The Book of Feeling Blue

Understand and Overcome Depression

Gwendoline Smith

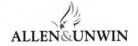

ALLEN&UNWIN

First published in Australia and New Zealand in 2023 by Allen & Unwin.

First Published in paperback in Great Britain in 2023 by
Allen & Unwin, an imprint of Atlantic Books Ltd.

Text copyright © Gwendoline Smith, 2023

Illustrations copyright © Georgia Arnold and Gabrielle Maffey, 2023

10 9 8 7 6 5 4 3 2 1

A CIP catalogue record for this book is available from the British Library.

Paperback ISBN: 978 1 83895 815 2
E-book ISBN: 978 1 83895 816 9

Design by Megan van Staden
Diagrams by Megan van Staden
Set in Galaxie Copernicus and Avenir

Printed in Great Britain by Clays Ltd, Elcograf S.p.A.

Allen & Unwin
An imprint of Atlantic Books Ltd
Ormond House
26–27 Boswell Street
London
WC1N 3JZ

www.allenandunwin.com/uk

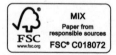

Most people assume it must be very painful
for me to remember being crazy.

It's not true.

Part of the pleasure I derive from my
memories comes from how much I appreciate
being sane now.

— Gwendoline Smith

CONTENTS

PART TWO

INTRODUCTION

The purpose of Part One of *The Book of Feeling Blue* is to provide you with information about whether you are experiencing a dose of 'the blues' or whether you are experiencing depression, and what sort of help is available. It also aims to provide you with some understanding of the strengths and pitfalls of the various treatment approaches. Part Two looks at how depression affects different groups in society, and the variety of approaches to managing it.

I am a great believer, as a mental health clinician, in providing people with as much education as I am able. I believe there are a number of benefits from this 'psychoeducation': it works not only to inform but also to demystify and destigmatise all forms of mental illness, not just depression.

Demystification breaks down the layers of superstitious beliefs about these illnesses, as well as the 'black magic' theories about psychiatric treatments and the scepticism within certain faith communities regarding secular (non-religious) psychotherapy or medical approaches.

Destigmatisation is a by-product of having scientifically based information. This takes away the shame from both the diagnosis and the process of asking for help. It also enables families to ask for support from their extended families and communities when caring for a family member with a mental illness or mood disorder.

PART
ONE

CHAPTER ONE

FEELING BLUE

From the late 1300s, the expression 'feeling blue' has been used to mean being sad. But there are many other cultural meanings given to the colour blue. In Western countries, blue also denotes safety and trust or authority; for example, the blue uniforms worn by the police. It has also been linked with masculinity — that old notion 'blue is for boys, pink for girls' — and associated with tranquillity.

- In Indian culture it is associated with Lord Krishna, and represents bravery and strength.
- In Latin America it represents hope, but also mourning.
- In Chinese culture, blue symbolises immortality and advancement, and the season of spring.
- For Māori, blue is associated with the sky father, Ranginui.

Universally, the associations of the colour blue are primarily positive. However, in Western contemporary culture the colour blue also has a strong association with sadness.

In Africa, blue is the colour of harmony and love, symbolising the importance of peace and togetherness. Yet for the African people who were taken to the New World to work as slaves, singing 'the blues' was something different again. These were songs of their despair and suffering, sung to make the time pass more quickly. Historians refer to blues music as being about the slaves' struggle to survive and their efforts to win back their freedom. Perhaps our collective consciousness of 'feeling blue' also emanates partly from our resonance with the universal language of music such as the blues.

FEELING SAD

Sadness is something all of us experience. You might feel sad because someone has died, because a relationship has ended, because you have experienced a loss of some kind, any kind — a friend, a job, an opportunity.

Feeling sad or 'blue' is very much a part of our emotional repertoire. You feel happy sometimes;

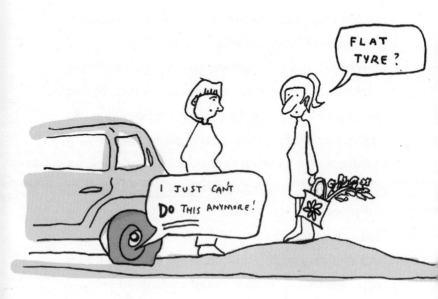

and at other times you feel disappointed; you feel angry, excited or frustrated; you feel blue.

Emotions are innate. They are biologically driven reactions to certain challenges and opportunities, sculpted by evolution to help humans survive, as part of the 'fight/flight/freeze' response.

Some emotions, such as shame and guilt, are learned emotions, shaped by the social and cultural environment we grow up in.

What I have observed in my clinical work, particularly in the past twenty or so years, is that if we don't like how we experience an emotion, we don't want it to be there. If you happen to be feeling sad about the breakdown of your relationship, you might find yourself surrounded by people making comments such as 'You'll get over it', 'Snap out of it', 'Think positively'.

Although your friends and loved ones are trying to be helpful, this pressure to never feel sad or 'blue' is very rarely helpful. These comments also tend to encourage people to suppress feelings that are a part of being human.

Poets often describe pain and joy as two sides of the same coin — both are necessary for a life that is fully lived. An example is John Keats' 'Ode on Melancholy' written in 1819.

PRESSURE TO BE HAPPY

The world that you are living in endlessly sends you messages that you not only *should* be happy but also *deserve* to be happy. Everywhere you look, people's social media profiles are immaculately curated to show their happiest selves.

Billions of dollars are spent showing you what products to buy to be truly happy — the foods, fashions, cosmetic surgery, cars, holidays . . . an endless supply of things and stuff that will ensure you never have to feel blue. Of course, the other inference here is that if you do feel 'blue' and dissatisfied you must be a loser who can't afford what it takes to be an always-happy winner, with a happy, perfect life.

When the fact is . . .

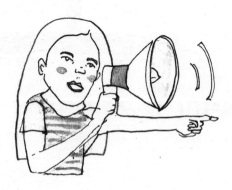

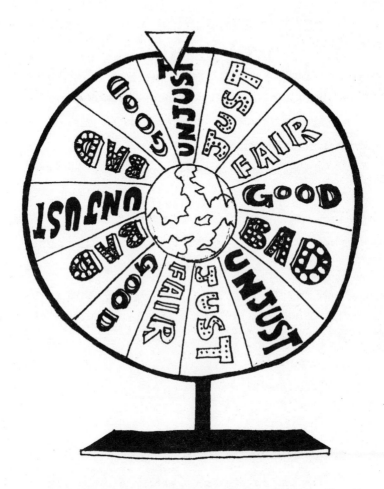

REALITY IS RANDOM AND CHANCE

What's more, as I wrote in my earlier book *The Book of Knowing*:

If you don't accept reality for what it is, you're f@#ked. Because the universe doesn't care. It is not just nor is it fair. Otherwise, bad things wouldn't happen to good people.

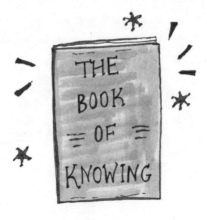

In this same context, I do not believe in the word *deserve*. You do not deserve to feel sad after a loss or traumatic event, you just are. It is not a punishment.

Sometimes you might feel sad or blue because of things that are happening in your world. What is important is how you find your way to the other side.

THE MYTH OF 'MAKE ME'

Another important fact to understand is that no one can *make you* feel sad or blue. Other people may impact on or influence your emotional state, but you are ultimately responsible for how you feel (unless of course it is caused by something biological like the flu, a stomach bug, a broken limb, depression, etc.).

In *The Book of Angst* I draw attention to this phenomenon. It sounds something like this:

'He made me feel sad/blue.'
'She made me feel angry.'
'They made me feel worthless.'
**THESE STATEMENTS
ARE NOT TRUE!**

How you think about yourself and your world creates how you feel. Sure, you can be influenced by factors in your environment, but ultimately it's all your work. (That is, unless the 'feeling blue' morphs into being depressed, and your biology starts to take hold — more on that later.)

It may feel as though the emotions you are experiencing are independent of you and are being inflicted upon you by the world, but that quite simply is not true. Think about it this way (from *The Book of Angst*):

> *I can't make you love me, I can't make you smile or cry — you do that. If someone you love doesn't love you back, you may feel sad and blue but you don't get to change it. Likewise, if you don't want to establish an intimate relationship with someone they can't make you.*

THE LOCUS OF CONTROL

You may not have heard of this term. It refers to the extent to which you feel as though you have control over the events and influences in your life, and therefore how you manage them. If you constantly look outside of yourself for happiness and fulfilment — through things like consumables, other people, religion or money — you never learn how to trust your own abilities and develop your own resilience.

In fact, we all operate according to what psychologists refer to as this locus of control. It relates to an individual's perception about the underlying main causes of events in their life. So, in other words, are you in control of your own destiny (internal locus of control), or do you believe that you are controlled by external forces such as fate or God or other people (external locus of control)?

I encourage the belief that the locus of control needs to be internal. This means *you* get to choose. The external pursuit of happiness positions you as a victim, or, as I often say: 'You live like a leaf in the wind.' If you can be destabilised by the slightest breeze, you'll never be prepared for the inevitable storms that life will dish out.

RECENT RESEARCH

Interestingly, researchers have now shown that allowing yourself to experience 'not-so-happy' feelings develops resilience, hence promoting psychological wellbeing. One research team found that the link between negative mental states and poor emotional and physical health was weaker

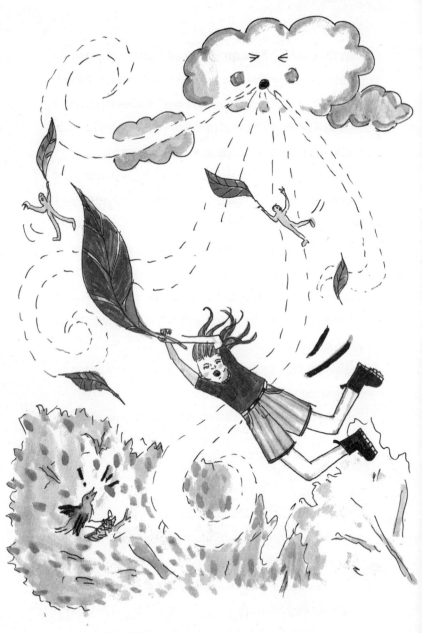

If you have an external locus of control, you can end up living like a leaf in the wind.

in individuals who considered negative moods as useful. Indeed, negative moods correlated with low life satisfaction only in people who did not perceive adverse feelings as helpful or pleasant (Luong, Wrzus, Wagner & Riedeger, *Emotion*, 2016).

Other cross-cultural studies also indicate that people living in Westernised countries are four to ten times more likely to experience depression and anxiety than people from cultures where both positive and negative emotions are considered to be an essential part of life. In such cultures there does not appear to be the same constant pressure to be happy and joyful.

It is interesting to note, however, that in Eastern cultures that have become heavily Westernised, such as Japan, mood disturbance has increased, as have suicide rates.

HAPPINESS ENTITLEMENT

The Baby Boomers (born 1946–64) have never really suffered the hardship their parents had on a societal scale, living through world wars and severe economic depression.

Neither have their children:

- Gen X: born 1965–80
- Gen Y: born 1981–96
- Gen Z: born 1997–2012

For these generations, happiness and pleasure are viewed as a 'given' or a 'right'. Hardship is an inconvenience, and something that can be fixed by the parental figure. This teaches them the big golden myth: 'Thou shalt never, and never have to, experience discomfort.'

The Baby Boomers remembered the suffering and hardship experienced by their parents, and vowed and declared that their children's lives would be different. However, although this seems to be a magnanimous belief system, it actually risks teaching entitlement, and can result in the lowering of discomfort tolerance.

Being able to tolerate discomfort is essential for resilience. A child who can adapt to all weathers is equipped to deal with frustration, disappointment, loss, unfairness and injustice. The entitled prince and princess do not have these skills.

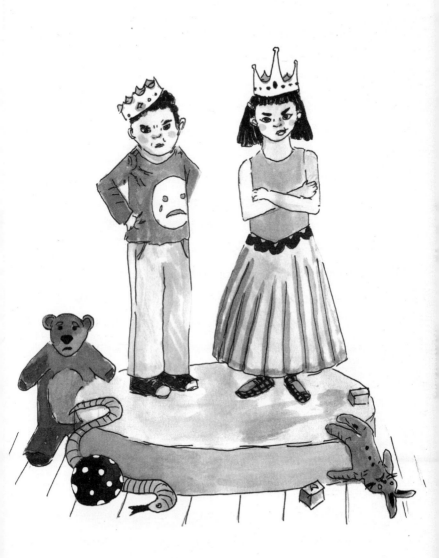

Here's a quote I really like, from American science fiction writer Robert A. Heinlein:

Don't handicap your children by making their lives easy.

Parents, particularly those with excessive wealth, can protect their children from certain hardships. But you can never protect them from death and rejection or illnesses like Covid. These are random life events which we all experience, and from which no amount of money and indulgence can protect us.

THE COVID BLUES

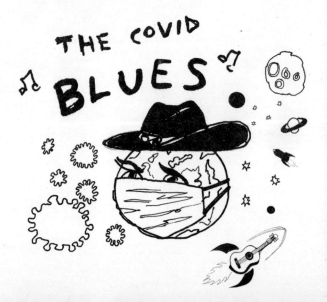

Just before we leave the subject of entitlement, one of the things I observed, particularly in the first wave of the Covid pandemic, was a real sense of being inconvenienced.

- 'What do you mean we can't go on our overseas trip?'
- 'I hate not being able to go out to clubs or have parties with three hundred of my closest friends!'
- 'I *shouldn't* have to wear a mask or have a vaccine. I *should* be able to do what I want, not what "they" [of course, there's always a "they"] want me to do!'

There was frequently a sense of 'They have no right to dictate to us what we *should* and *shouldn't* be able to do!'

Should and should not are popular mantras of the entitled!

However, as time progressed and the death toll rose, the landscape changed. The pandemic swept uncaringly, unfairly and unjustly across the world. Very real mental health issues began to emerge —

an epidemic of fear and worry on a global scale, particularly among certain groups such as the elderly, care providers and people with underlying health conditions.

Rates of anxiety soared across all age groups and in many different forms: health anxiety, worry (generalised anxiety), OCD (obsessive compulsive disorder). Young people began to experience more depression and anxiety. They had difficulty maintaining their motivation, and they felt powerlessness and pessimism about the future.

These phenomena can lead to both the blues and depression. In his work on 'learned helplessness', Martin Seligman highlights the profound psychological contribution that powerlessness, hopelessness and helplessness make to depression.

The Covid pandemic has confronted us all with these experiences, giving many of us what you might call 'the Covid blues'.

Tips for managing the Covid blues

It is impossible to predict where the world will be at with regard to the Covid pandemic and its psychological impact when this book goes to print and is released into bookshops. However, just in case we continue to be surprised by Covid's enduring capacity to metamorphose — or some other pandemic has come along — here are a few mental health tips based on advice from the World Health Organization.

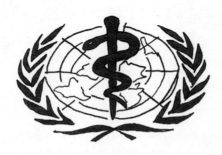

- Keep informed with information from trusted, **reputable** sources, but avoid over-exposure to information.
- Keep up with your daily routines as much as possible. Combine work with exercise and doing enjoyable things. Don't spend too much time in your pyjamas — although I know that habit to be seductive, especially in the winter months.
- Combat isolation by staying in touch with others by telephone or through online channels, especially family members overseas or far away.

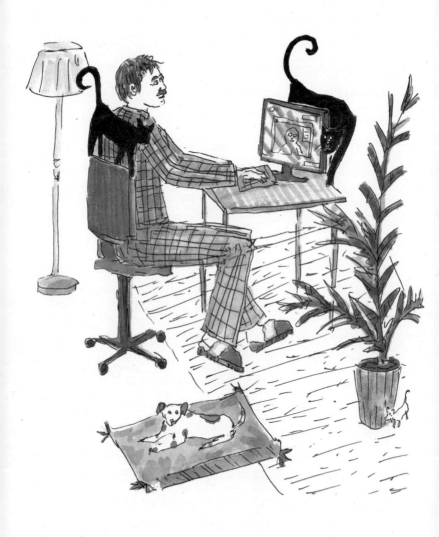

Keep up with your daily routines — and try to avoid
spending too much time in your pyjamas!

- Be mindful of alcohol and substance consumption.
- Watch the amount of screentime you engage in per day, avoiding long periods of time spent playing video games and scrolling Instagram.
- Be kind to other people and see if there are ways you can support others (for example, helping with online shopping).
- If you are a worrier, or finding yourself worrying more since the arrival of Covid, have a look at my book on overthinking (couldn't resist that opportunity).

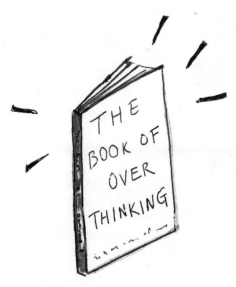

WHAT TO DO IF YOU'RE JUST FEELING 'BLUE'

I'd just like to emphasise that in this chapter I am referring to strategies for the blues, which is not to be confused with depression. When you have the 'blues', you probably feel sad, tearful and withdrawn, with a lack of energy or motivation. These feelings tend to be mild and will pass without causing too much disruption to your daily routine. These phases of sadness are very much a part of everyday life.

Feeling blue or a bit down every now and then can provide you with a little tap on the shoulder to remind you to look at areas of your life that may need changing. The blues don't just appear 'out of the blue'. They are more often associated with something specific (for example, disappointment, relationship breakdown, loss, frustration or betrayal).

How you can shift the blues

You can often lighten your mood by the simplest of interventions.

- Spend time with loved ones.
- Watch a favourite funny show.

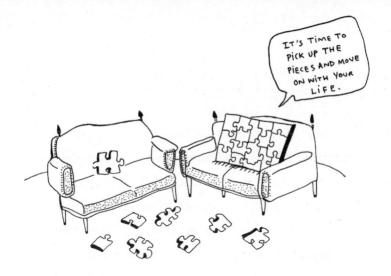

- Focus on a pastime or hobby. I find jigsaw puzzles quite hypnotic and good for distracting me from my woes.
- Talk through your feelings with someone — if not a friend then perhaps a therapist. Cognitive therapy offers an excellent problem–solution-focused approach.
- Get physically active. Go for a walk. Nature will always soothe a troubled soul. If the weather is nasty, watch a David Attenborough documentary.
- Do something creative: journal, draw, scrapbook, do some colouring, listen to music.
- Take the opportunity to do things that are out of your comfort zone.

AND FINALLY, THE 'WINTER BLUES'

The 'winter blues' are very common in parts of the world that experience long winters with very little sunlight. Technically this is referred to as SAD (seasonal affective disorder). In these countries, sufferers are commonly treated with light therapy boxes, but professional guidance is recommended.

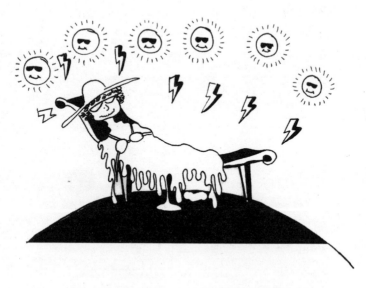

LIGHT THERAPY

CHAPTER TWO

BEYOND THE BLUES

Having had severe depression and breast cancer, depression in my experience was far worse. With breast cancer, I was in physical pain, but not the psychic pain of depression that prevented me from enjoying and living my life.

— Gwendoline Smith, *Breast Support*

A LOOK FROM THE INSIDE

As well as being a clinical psychologist, I am also in the one in a hundred individuals diagnosed with bipolar disorder or, as I prefer to call it, manic depression. I have spent many years of my adult life both working clinically with people with depression and managing my own manic-depressive episodes.

I would like to tell you a bit about my subjective experience of depression. If you have bought this book for yourself, it may take away some of the feelings of isolation you might be experiencing. If you have bought it to better understand what a loved one is going through, hopefully this inside look will help further your understanding of what exactly depression is like, and how you can be of help.

My story

I am a self-proclaimed extrovert. I love being stimulated by witty debate, conversation and humour, usually around a dinner table.

Yet, when I am depressed, there is no colour in anything. I can't digest food, let alone prepare a dinner party. I can't converse with anybody, not even those closest to me.

I had my first depressive episode in 1994, after a manic episode during which I had lived with the delusion of my being the Second Messiah (reincarnated as a female) for nearly a month. As you can imagine, there was a lot to be done — saving the planet being no small task, even before global warming became so apparent.

It was a wonderful and exhilarating experience. I enjoyed the sensation of travelling through space and time. (As a very dear colleague of mine, Professor Rob Kydd, once said, 'If you could bottle

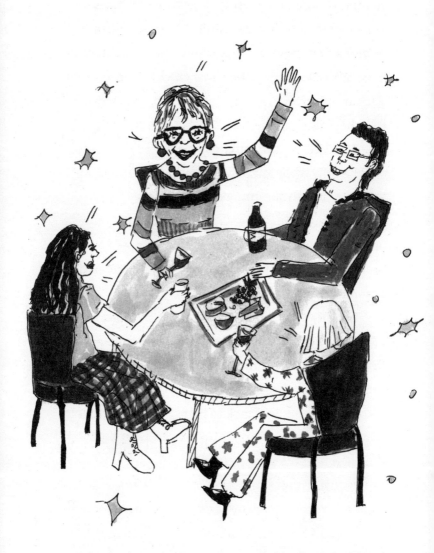

As an extrovert, I love dinner parties and social events. But when I'm depressed, I withdraw from the things that usually give me pleasure.

mania as a designer drug, you'd make a fortune.')
I also lived with the delusion that I was Elizabeth
Taylor's first daughter, the result of her torrid affair
with Walt Disney. At the same time I believed that
Richard Burton was my father, but I questioned
whether either of them was in fact my father, given
that I had been immaculately conceived.

The only question of any relevance was actually:
'When will she agree to take medication?'

My answer to that: 'I don't recall reading
anywhere that Jesus was prescribed lithium.'

I think you're starting to get the picture. Yes, I
was mad.

The only problem is that when you're high for so
long, eventually your chemicals will change and it
is time to come back down to earth. With the help of
antipsychotic medication, I did land, the delusions
dissipated and I was back to being a mere mortal.

Note: On the subject of antipsychotics, I know a lot of people perceive this type of medication in a very negative light, and are very wary of even a mention of these drugs being prescribed. In my opinion, this has a lot to do with the confusion between 'psychosis' and being a 'psychopath' — that having to take an antipsychotic is perceived to be the worst it can get, the lowest you can go; that you must be schizophrenic and untreatable; that you're on the verge of being locked up and the key thrown away. Having taken many antipsychotics over the years, I see them as *thought managers*. They help return delusional thoughts to a more rational reality — a very desirable outcome. They contribute a great deal in cases of manic psychosis, schizophrenia and drug-induced psychosis, and in small doses they help with intrusive, racing thoughts. Prescribed carefully, they are nothing to be afraid of.

After my mania was successfully treated, I then developed another inconvenient little condition, known in the trade as 'post-psychotic depression'. This particular ailment put me off work for another six months.

This was my first experience of depression. It flattened me like a steamroller. My confidence and self-belief were smashed. As a shell of my former self, I felt like I would never work again, laugh again, connect with people again.

As a clinician I had often witnessed the pain of depression on the faces of my clients, but never

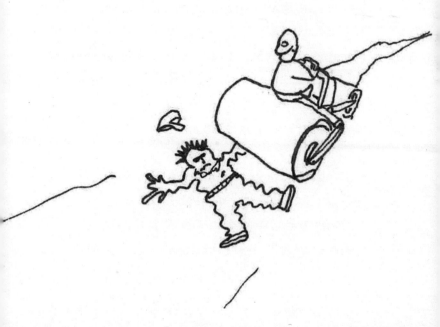

before had I come close to understanding the degree of debilitation, the intensity of the despair.

Really, only people who have experienced depression can truly understand what it is like. It is invisible to others and yet so frightening. It can be frustrating for loved ones, as there is no real evidence of 'illness' — a rash, blood, fever, a broken bone. However, it is my hope that as we demystify and destigmatise all mental illnesses, depression will benefit from this change in attitude.

On the subject of stigma, it is often thought of as something society, the community, friends and family are doing — expressing such sentiments as 'Just get over it'. But stigma is also internal. We seem to expect our brain to never get sick, to never feel strained. When it does, we get frustrated and impatient, and refuse to take time off work to recover, saying things like:

- 'I *should* be better by now', or
- 'I don't need help, I *should* be able to do this on my own. And I certainly do *not* need medication!!!'

However, depressive illness requires medication, while feeling blue does not. *One is an illness, the other is not.*

During my first episode of depression, I too was sceptical of medication and what it could offer. As a psychologist, I felt like such a failure having to 'resort to' medication to get well. Fortunately, however reluctant I was to take it, I responded well to an antidepressant medication.

As a clinician, I am very careful to separate feeling blue from clinical depression. Feeling blue is something that can be addressed through cognitive behavioural interventions, as well as environmental changes; for example, taking steps to resolve dysfunctional relationships or workplace bullying (to name just two).

However, once the manifestations of stress and strain continue to increase in number and severity, there is a significantly high probability that a depressive illness is the next landing strip . . .

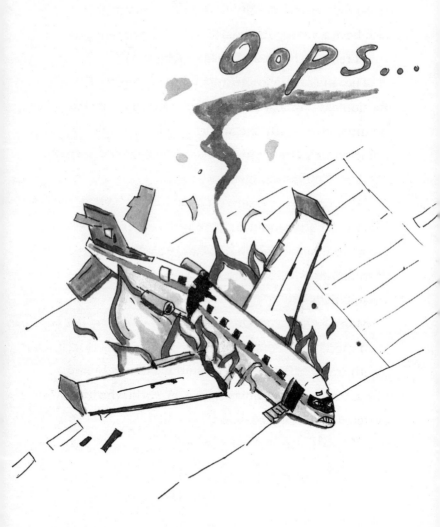

MELANCHOLIC DEPRESSION

Even today in the twenty-first century, many people still have a very archetypal image of depression. By that I refer to the idea of melancholia.

The melancholic depressive was depicted as motionless, almost vegetative, with no interest in interacting with the world or other people, as depicted in Vincent van Gogh's painting *Sorrowing Old Man (At Eternity's Gate)*.

Plagued by psychiatric illness throughout his life, van Gogh committed suicide in 1890. Evidence suggests that he had manic depression, a chronic mental illness that affects many creative people — myself included.

Many artists throughout history have struggled with mood disorders. Picasso had his blue period. Beethoven, Tchaikovsky, Leonard Cohen and Lady Gaga are but a few from the musical world who have suffered bouts of depression.

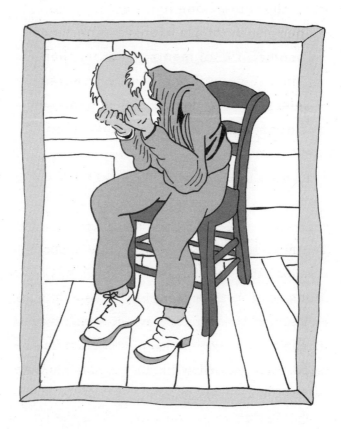

HOMAGE TO VAN GOGH'S
'SORROWING OLD MAN'

> **Note:** It's not that all creative people suffer from mental illness. It's just that out of one hundred creative people, more are likely to experience some form of mental disorder than in a sample of one hundred people selected at random. This has been well documented and widely discussed, but no one has come up with a definitive answer for why this is.

The first known use of the word melancholia to describe a disorder of mood came from the Greeks, in around 400 BC. More specifically, it was the Greek philosopher Hippocrates who concluded that the human body was composed of four main fluids — blood, black bile, yellow bile and phlegm — and that an imbalance of these could account for melancholia. I'm not quite convinced about the role of phlegm and bile in mental illness, but Hippocrates wasn't known as the 'Father of Medicine' for nothing. This was 400 BC and his 'Hippocratic Oath' still guides contemporary Western medicine.

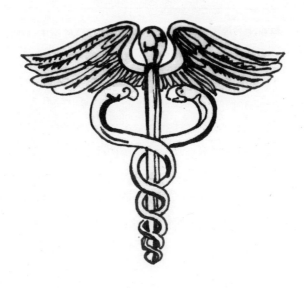

The Hippocratic Oath is often illustrated with the caduceus, a Western symbol of health and healing.

Hippocrates and other doctors worked on the assumption that all diseases had a natural cause rather than a 'supernatural' one. By contrast, priests believed that illnesses such as epilepsy were caused by the gods.

Psychiatric illness especially was surrounded by superstitious beliefs and the idea that it was based in black magic. In a religious or supernatural interpretation, conditions such as schizophrenia could be accounted for as a person being possessed by the devil or an evil spirit.

I love this definition from the *Merriam-Webster Dictionary*:

> *When disease was first used, it referred literally to 'lack of ease or comfort' rather than to how it is used today to refer to sickness or problems with bodily function. Disease can still be used today to mean 'uncomfortable,' but there is usually a hyphen as in 'dis-ease.'*

Think of it like a 'dissing of the ease'. When life moves too fast and we get stressed, when a relationship falls apart, when a loved one gets sick or dies, these events disturb the ease of our lives. We now refer to these difficult times and events as stressful, and there is no doubt in contemporary medicine that stress is capable of causing disease.

So if we drop the phlegm and the multicoloured bile, the Greeks were really on to something!

THE CHANGING FACE OF DEPRESSION: AGITATED DEPRESSION

I often describe agitated depression (AD) as the depressive illness of the twenty-first century. Agitated depression is considered to be a relatively severe type of clinical depression. It includes these classic features:

- persistent feelings of sadness/hopelessness
- pessimism/lack of enjoyment
- low energy
- inability to concentrate
- ongoing thoughts of death or suicide.

These symptoms are experienced in combination with agitated symptoms such as:

- irritability
- anxiety
- restlessness
- excessive talking
- fidgeting and/or angry outbursts.

The particularly unpleasant word to describe this phenomenon — when a medical condition is simultaneously present with one or more others — is *comorbidity*. The depression we tend to see most often as clinicians these days is this combination of depressive and agitated symptoms.

Hence, unlike what occurs with melancholia, individuals with agitated depression continue to function, but they become increasingly stressed, their sleep becomes disturbed and their appetite fluctuates significantly — more like what you would see with anxiety disorders.

Gender issues: the male perspective

I would like to make a couple of generalised comments about the men who I see clinically presenting with lowered mood/depression.

Firstly: they have usually been struggling for some time, often years.

Secondly: they rarely self-refer; they are usually metaphorically dragged along by their partners. The exception is when the untreated mood disorder has resulted in divorce/separation.

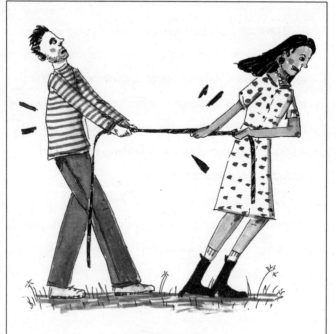

Early signs of depression in men can include an
increase in:

- anger
- frustration
- aggression
- irritability.

You will observe that this symptom list is far
more linked to agitated depression than to
melancholia.

These differences may be due to societal expectations of how men and women express emotion. It is likely that men are less willing to show certain emotions, such as sadness, if they feel that others may judge or criticise them for it. They may also view experiencing fear-based anxiety as weakness.

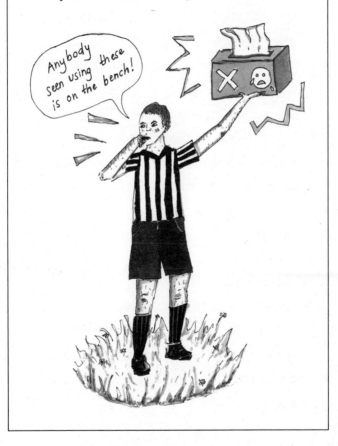

ANXIETY AND DEPRESSION

You may be wondering, if there is such a close relationship between anxiety and depression, what comes first? Does one cause the other? No need to phone a friend. I'll give you the answer.

> The relationship between anxiety and depression is very much 'chicken and egg'.

Let me elaborate. Anxiety conditions such as generalised anxiety (worry), fear of judgement (social anxiety) and post-traumatic stress disorder (PTSD) can place so much strain on a person's system that a depression results. Likewise, people with depression can become socially withdrawn and begin to worry and think more pessimistically. Confused? I would be if I were you!

So anxiety can cause depression, and depression can cause anxiety. Hence, does the chicken come first, or the egg?

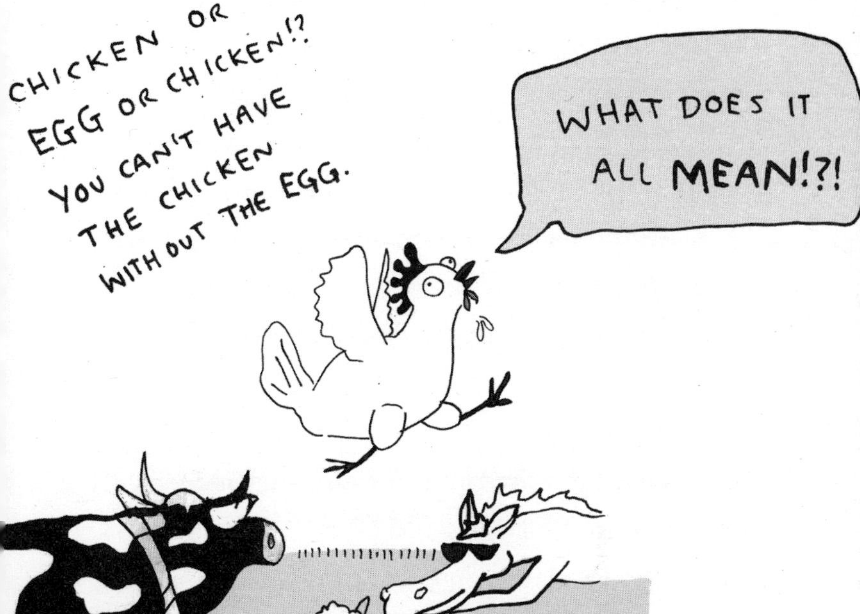
CHICKEN OR EGG OR CHICKEN!? YOU CAN'T HAVE THE CHICKEN WITH OUT THE EGG.
WHAT DOES IT ALL MEAN!?!

The answer is that, more often than not, the anxiety comes first, then as the system begins to collapse the depression turns up. (The exception to this would be PTSD, where a person can have no pre-existing anxiety or depression but start to experience it following a traumatic event.)

In fact, the link between anxiety and depression exists within a very complex neurological system. The diagram below explains the mechanics of the stress response, and how an adaptive (survival) response can become a maladaptive response that serves no useful purpose.

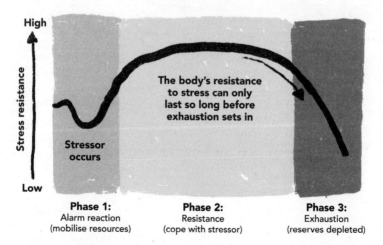

General Adaptation Syndrome (GAS)
(Identified by Hans Selye in 1936)

The body's resistance to stress can only last so long before exhaustion sets in

Stressor occurs

Stress resistance — High / Low

Phase 1:
Alarm reaction
(mobilise resources)

Phase 2:
Resistance
(cope with stressor)

Phase 3:
Exhaustion
(reserves depleted)

Our stress response system defends, then fatigues.

Then there are hormones to consider. They keep us afloat by producing adrenaline and cortisol. But if they are active in the system over prolonged periods of time, their presence can begin to erode the immune system.

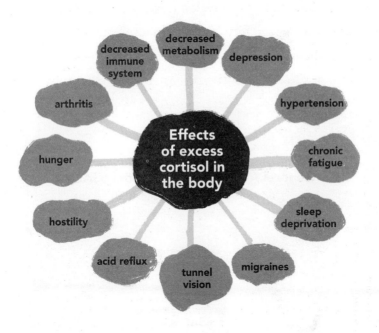

I describe stress hormones as being like Voltaren, that wonderful anti-inflammatory most of us are familiar with. If, say, we have an injured leg, we take

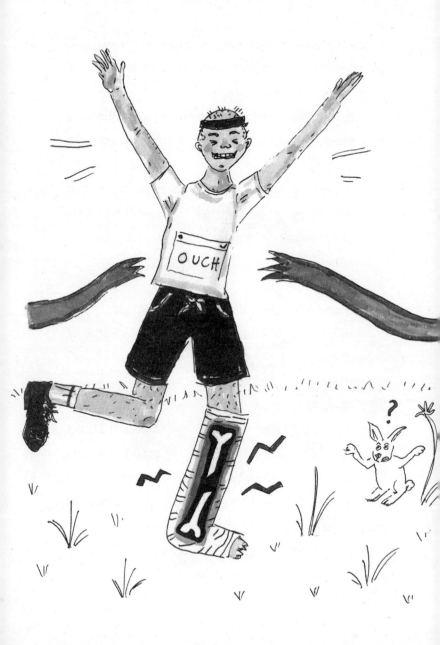

the pill or plaster on the gel, and with the use of this temporary crutch, life goes on at the same speed as ever — no sore leg!

But, of course, payback time comes the following day, when your leg is hurting so much that you can hardly walk!

Have you ever noticed that the night before you are about to go on holiday, after working furiously to get everything done before departure, you feel a tickle in the back of your throat? Sure enough, on the way to the airport, you find yourself stopping off for lozenges, cough mixture and nasal spray.

Why? Well, the neurotransmitters in charge of thinking about the holiday and what type of energy is required start sending out messages to the troops. *Hey, team, she's off on holiday. No more need for you stress hormones to keep producing. It's been a bloody tough year, what with Covid and everything that goes with that. So take a break for a couple of weeks!*

And yes, it's as simple as that: a systemic change manifesting in flu-like symptoms.

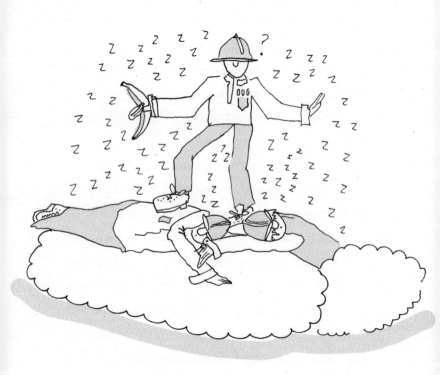

When your stress hormones finally get to take a break . . .

WHAT ABOUT GRIEF?

Good question!

After significant loss, humans and many other species of animals grieve. We've all heard the stories of dogs sitting at their owners' grave sites or returning to the place where they died. I love those stories, but they're so sad. We as humans always feel the need to explain things, and we can't explain to a dog what has happened, but I suspect with their extraordinary senses they know their owner is gone and isn't coming back.

Grief is very much like the experience of depression. You might experience loss of appetite, lack of enjoyment of life, withdrawal, lack of energy. Both conditions look and often feel identical.

Grief-focused therapy, often in groups, can be exceptionally helpful, especially if the grief is a result of the tragic loss of a child. Only other people who have experienced this unimaginable loss are able to relate, even on a non-verbal level.

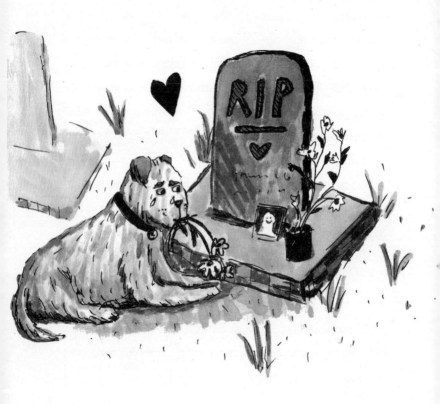

Did you know that there is no word in the English language for someone who has lost a child? If a woman loses her spouse she is a widow, if a man loses his spouse he is a widower, if a child loses their parents they are an orphan. Don't ask me why — I can only think that such a horrifying thought or experience dared not be acknowledged formally in the English language. Or perhaps it has to do with the limitation of English when it comes to describing emotions on a very deep level. For example, our friends the Ancient Greeks had seven words to describe the different stages and types of love. Sanskrit, the ancient Indo-European language of India, takes the lead with ninety-six different words!

In certain parts of the world, the word vilomah is gaining acceptance to describe a parent who has lost a child. Vilomah comes from the Sanskrit language, which also gave us the word 'widow', meaning empty.

When people present to my clinic with grief, they are usually experiencing depressive-like symptoms, and the subjective experience — how they feel and act — can often be the same as if they were experiencing depression.

What I point out is that if grief dominates mood and outlook for more than two to four weeks, it is likely that the natural sadness around grief has morphed into depression — the chemicals in the body have changed and the sadness has developed into a clinical phenomenon.

After careful consideration, I'll then discuss the contribution that medication has to offer. It may not be appropriate to treat the pain being suffered, especially by a vilomah, with medication. However, this should not be discounted, as this is a profoundly painful experience.

CHAPTER THREE

HOW TO TELL THE DIFFERENCE BETWEEN THE BLUES AND DEPRESSION

B efore we discuss this, have a look at this model. It will help you understand a great deal about how lowered mood impacts on our totality. It is genius in its simplicity.

The model illustrates definitively the *interconnectedness* of all aspects of ourselves: our biology, behaviour, emotion and cognition (thought), and how these interact with our environment.

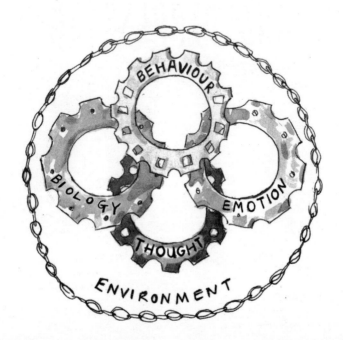

I have intentionally used the word 'inter-connectedness', as essentially we are not a whole lot of parts joined together. Gabor Maté, a fabulous world-renowned physician, points out that all of evolution is based on the initial construction of a single-celled organism. Then the one cell becomes a multi-celled organism. Then the different cells move about and become specialised cells — the digestive system, the senses, the brain, etc. — all the while maintaining the same DNA. Yet we are all created from one cell, one sperm, one egg.

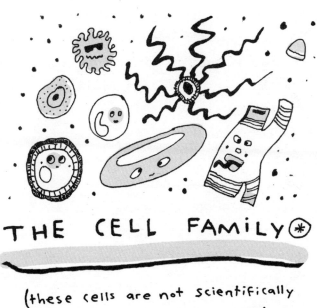

THE CELL FAMILY✳

(these cells are not scientifically accurate, just very cute ♥)

However, for the purposes of therapy, compartmentalising — as per the model — allows us to describe how we work, and how all these aspects of ourselves are interrelated. Depression intrudes upon all of these domains.

BECK'S DEPRESSION INVENTORY

One of the first things I will do in an initial appointment with a new patient is assess whether or not someone is stressed, distressed, feeling blue, or depressed. I determine this by administering 'Beck's Depression Inventory' (see opposite). This scale is internationally used and respected. The designer of the inventory, Aaron Beck, is recognised to be the founding father of cognitive therapy as it is practised today.

Beck's Depression Inventory is also designed to account for variations in the biological, behavioural, emotional and cognitive (thought-based) aspects of our lives (as per the diagram on page 66).

The inventory can be self-scored, just by totalling up your scores. If you wish you can do it online and have it scored for you.

Beck's Depression Inventory

Circle your responses to the following questions:

Q1.

0   I do not feel sad.

1   I feel sad.

2   I am sad all the time and I can't snap out of it.

3   I am so sad and unhappy that I can't stand it.

Q2.

0   I am not particularly discouraged about
    the future.

1   I feel discouraged about the future.

2   I feel I have nothing to look forward to.

3   I feel the future is hopeless and that things
    cannot improve.

Q3.

0   I do not feel like a failure.

1   I feel I have failed more than the average
    person.

2   As I look back on my life, all I can see is a lot
    of failures.

3   I feel I am a complete failure as a person.

Q4.

0   I get as much satisfaction out of things as
    I used to.

1   I don't enjoy things the way I used to.

2   I don't get satisfaction out of anything anymore.

3   I am dissatisfied or bored with everything.

Q5.

0   I don't feel particularly guilty.

1   I feel guilty a good part of the time.

2   I feel quite guilty most of the time.

3   I feel guilty all of the time.

Q6.

0   I don't feel I am being punished.

1   I feel I may be punished.

2   I expect to be punished.

3   I feel I am being punished.

Q7.

0   I don't feel disappointed in myself.

1   I am disappointed in myself.

2   I am disgusted with myself.

3   I hate myself.

Q8.

0   I don't feel I am any worse than anybody else.

1   I am critical of myself for my weaknesses or mistakes.

2   I blame myself all the time for my faults.

3   I blame myself for everything bad that happens.

Q9.

0   I don't have any thoughts of killing myself.

1   I have thoughts of killing myself, but I would not carry them out.

2   I would like to kill myself.

3   I would kill myself if I had the chance.

Q10.

0   I don't cry any more than usual.

1   I cry more now than I used to.

2   I cry all the time now.

3   I used to be able to cry, but now I can't cry even though I want to.

Q11.

0   I am no more irritated by things than
    I ever was.

1   I am slightly more irritated now than usual.

2   I am quite annoyed or irritated a good deal
    of the time.

3   I feel irritated all the time.

Q12.

0   I have not lost interest in other people.

1   I am less interested in other people than
    I used to be.

2   I have lost most of my interest in other
    people.

3   I have lost all of my interest in other people.

Q13.

0   I make decisions about as well as I ever
    could.

1   I put off making decisions more than
    I used to.

2   I have greater difficulty in making decisions
    than I used to.

3   I can't make decisions at all anymore.

Q14.

0   I don't feel that I look any worse than
    I used to.

1   I am worried that I am looking old or
    unattractive.

2   I feel there are permanent changes in my
    appearance that make me look unattractive.

3   I believe that I look ugly.

Q15.

0   I can work about as well as before.

1   It takes an extra effort to get started at doing
    something.

2   I have to push myself very hard to do
    anything.

3   I can't do any work at all.

Q16.

0   I can sleep as well as usual.

1   I don't sleep as well as I used to.

2   I wake up 1–2 hours earlier than usual and
    find it hard to get back to sleep.

3   I wake up several hours earlier than I used to
    and cannot get back to sleep.

Q17.

0   I don't get more tired than usual.

1   I get tired more easily than I used to.

2   I get tired from doing almost anything.

3   I am too tired to do anything.

Q18.

0   My appetite is no worse than usual.

1   My appetite is not as good as it used to be.

2   My appetite is much worse now.

3   I have no appetite at all anymore.

Q19.

0   I haven't lost much weight, if any, lately.

1   I have lost more than five pounds.

2   I have lost more than ten pounds.

3   I have lost more than fifteen pounds.

Q20.

0   I am no more worried about my health than usual.

1   I am worried about physical problems like
    aches, pains, upset stomach or constipation.

2   I am very worried about physical problems
    and it's hard to think of much else.

3 I am so worried about my physical problems that I cannot think of anything else.

Q21.

0 I have not noticed any recent change in my interest in sex.

1 I am less interested in sex than I used to be.

2 I have almost no interest in sex.

3 I have lost interest in sex completely.

Once you have completed the questionnaire, add up the score for each of the 21 questions. The highest possible total for the whole test would be 63. The lowest possible score for the test would be zero.

Total score	Level of depression
1–10	These ups and downs are considered normal
11–16	Mild mood disturbance
17–20	Borderline clinical depression
21–30	Moderate depression
31–40	Severe depression
over 40	Extreme depression

If you or your loved one have crossed into the upper end of the scale, the approach to treatment is very different to what would be applied if you have a low score. Let's go through the scale together so you can understand it with more clarity, and are able to interpret the ranges and levels of depression you or your loved one may be experiencing.

Score of 1-10

Normal ups and downs — parking ticket, stubbed toe, broken fingernail. Shit happens! Frustration, and maybe, if they all happen on the same day, very mild blues.

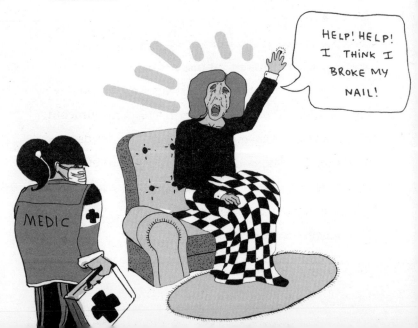

Score of 11 -16

Mild mood disturbance. Often in this range is someone starting to experience the impact of burnout at work. Problems in the family might be causing significant distress — issues with your teenagers, or in-fighting with your siblings over the division of the family assets after the death of a parent.

This could still fit under the classification of 'the blues', but is heading towards more of a frustrated and agitated response.

Score of 17 - 20

The borderline for a clinical depression. Things are starting to look quite a bit more serious.

Along with all of the unpleasantness in your day-to-day life, your body is starting to communicate that there are problems in your personal landscape that need to be resolved. You are also getting a message that if you don't change something soon you're going to pay the price, physically, emotionally and psychologically.

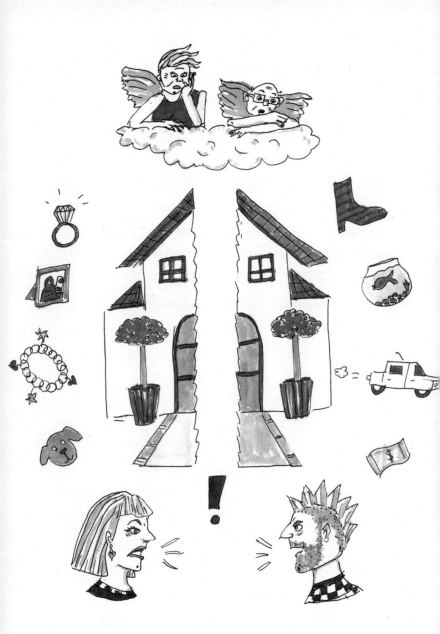

Problems in the family, such as disputes over property, can cause significant distress. This might lead to a mild mood disturbance.

Your gut is starting to play up. (If you would like to learn more about the role of the gut and the brain in depression and anxiety, google Harriet Brown's 2005 article in the *New York Times*, 'A brain in the head, and one in the gut'.)

You're more irritable and more fatigued, and your sleep is no longer refreshing. You feel exhausted and your enjoyment of life is rapidly decreasing, but you still manage to get up and face the demands of the day — just.

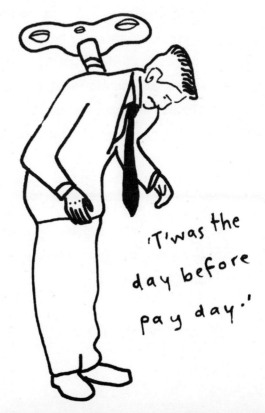

'Twas the day before pay day.'

Score of 21-30

Now we're into the big league.

When a score sits between 21 and 26 I am happy to work with psychological therapy only. However, above that the depressive illness has taken hold and medication is required. Before psychological therapy can even begin to be effective, medication is necessary.

Large numbers of people continue to function at this level. However, life is feeling increasingly futile, and everything is becoming a chore. You have to work harder than normal because your concentration, attention span and decision-making abilities are becoming impaired.

These psychological functions are known as executive temporal lobe functions. They are both sophisticated and fragile. Hence, even with a mild/moderate depression they will start to struggle. They are inevitably the first systems to shut down and the last brain functions to return to a normal level of functioning.

While I am happy to begin psychological therapy without medication at a score below 26 — sometimes

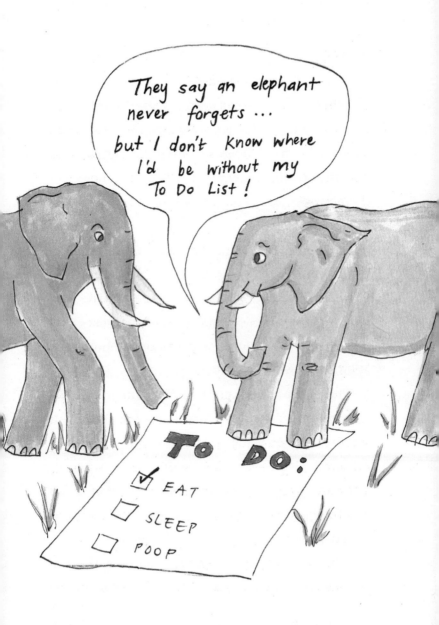

adjusting people's environmental and interpersonal conditions can lift a depression, even at this level — I will place a caveat on how long the standalone, psychologically based therapeutic relationship can continue before I strongly suggest the use of medication. Just like my psychiatrist had to do with me. It went a bit like this:

As I mentioned, once I had returned to earth after my manic episode, the depression I experienced was so severe I couldn't eat and I rarely got out of bed. I had lost an excessive amount of weight and was looking gaunt. However, my view at the time was closer to Patsy in *Absolutely Fabulous*, whose philosophy was: you can never have too many hats, gloves and shoes — and you can never be too thin.

My psychiatrist, Margaret Honeyman, did not adhere to that sentiment, however, and I must admit I was so depressed that I never got to appreciate being thin. Margaret gave me two weeks to get my shit together by whatever means — self-help, natural alternatives, diet and exercise routines. Believe me, I tried all of them.

If I returned at the end of that time with no apparent progress, it was MEDICATION TIME!

I felt as if I had failed as both a human and a psychologist — but I was to be proved wrong.

Score of 31-40

Severe depression. There is now no bargaining about whether medical treatments are required. Gone are the days of St John's wort and Rescue Remedy. At this level the depression is debilitating, and often may require hospitalisation, as suicidal thoughts will be increasing in frequency and intensity.

You are clinically depressed, but with the right medication, family support, rest, and community mental health and individual psychological support it is possible to make it through.

A few vital things to do at this stage:

1. Contact your doctor. (Although you probably already have.)
2. Take time off work. (Your doctor will provide a medical certificate for you.)
3. If you have loss-of-income insurance, activate that immediately, as you may have a stand-down period to start with.

Score Over 40

As a clinician in private practice, it is rare that I will meet someone this ill. The family will be well aware of the depression's severity, and often will have contacted private and community-based clinicians.

Hospitalisation, although undesirable (and I speak from experience, having been committed a number of times), is often the only way to keep someone safe. It is an awful decision to make when it involves a loved one, but this is when you really need to remember that you are not a mental health professional.

Often by this stage, as above, suicidal thoughts will be frequent and attempts may have started.

These very severe depressions can often evolve this way into a psychotic depression.

Psychotic depression is a subtype of major depression, and it occurs when a severe depressive illness includes some form of psychosis. This might be hallucinations (such as hearing voices telling you that you are a bad person), delusions (such as intense feelings of failure or worthlessness), or some other break with reality.

According to WebMD, psychotic depression affects around 25 per cent of people admitted to hospital for depression.

Psychotic depression is rare and very severe, but it can occur, particularly in people who refuse to seek professional help.

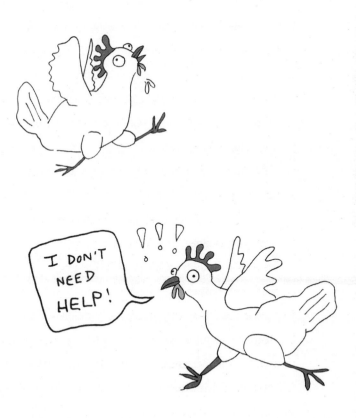

Is it any wonder . . . ?

One of the things I find most intriguing about the world I practise in is some people's reluctance and often refusal to accept professional medical help. But perhaps this is not surprising when you think about the process involved in being hospitalised with mental health issues.

Think about it: You have a loved one with a severe psychiatric illness, and they have become a danger to themselves and possibly others. To intervene, you have to make the ghastly decision to have them committed. You organise two assessing psychiatrists, sign the paperwork (feeling like Judas) and watch your loved one get taken away by the police.

Now let's flick channels and go over to the world of 'proper' medicine. Can you imagine someone having to be taken by the police for their chemotherapy session?

Or someone who has been waiting for a knee operation for two years, now limping through life in pain, having to be restrained to go for surgery. WTF is up with that!?

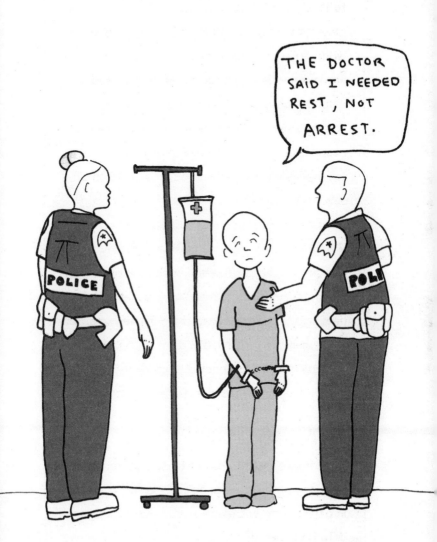

WHAT CAUSES DEPRESSION?

By now you will have discovered whether or not there is depression in your life, either your own or a loved one's. So let's have a look at some of the potential causes.

It is important to emphasise at this point that it is rare that a single reason can be pinpointed as the cause of depression. It tends to be the result of a number of contributing factors:

Heredity

The research is clear that some people have a genetic predisposition for depression. However, a susceptibility does not mean you will absolutely suffer depressive illness in your lifetime. What it can mean is that your genetic capacity to tolerate stress is lower, and hence your risk is increased.

Biochemistry

This is inextricably linked to the genetic theory above. The more science tells us about the human brain, the more we understand that our mood is mediated by electrical activity and certain chemicals within the brain. Dopamine — pleasure. Serotonin

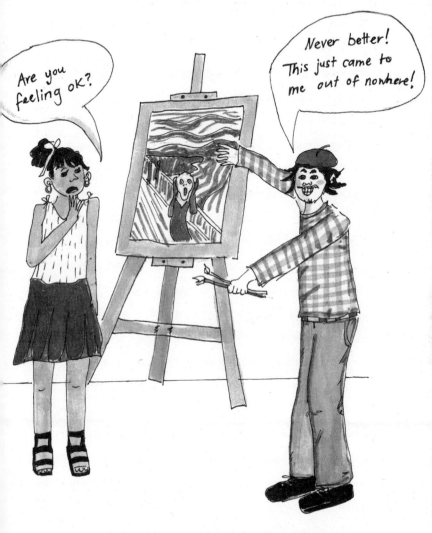

Depression is linked to our biochemistry. It's not just an abstract concept that exists outside of us.

— mood elevation. Endorphins — nice buzz.

You see, despair is not some poetic and abstract concept through which we feel love, pain and passion, nor one which we can paint and write poems and songs about, almost as though it exists outside of us.

No, ladies and gentlemen, it is all about our biology — our physical self. What we feel is maintained and established by our physical bodies.

Imagine this: you go to a light switch and turn the light on. Wait a minute . . . there's no light, because there is no power. Without power, the light won't switch on. There's no black magic or anything spooky there — just a basic fact.

Your body is just the same. You wake up and really want to welcome the day — but no chance, the power isn't on. You want to feel happy and interested in things again — fat chance. Why? Because you don't have the biochemicals you need to experience those things. The light won't go on because the power is off.

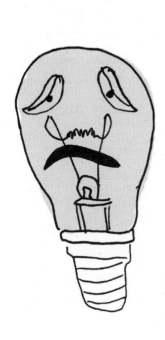

Physical considerations

Depression can sit alongside other physical illnesses. Other illnesses can also masquerade as depression (for example, thyroid problems, sleep apnoea, glandular fever). So it is important that your assessing clinician covers these possibilities prior to diagnosing depression.

So, as you may have gathered, depression is a complex condition in many ways. It is biologically, behaviourally and cognitively debilitating. Yet, as I mentioned earlier, resistance to psychiatric treatment is still alive and well across the globe. Why all the fuss?

CHAPTER FOUR

IMAGES OF PSYCHIATRY

efore I talk about the treatments available to you or your loved one, I would like to address further this reluctance so many people have when it comes to seeking help for mental health issues and/or from the mental health profession. This ongoing trepidation when it comes to psychiatric treatments emanates from a number of sources:

- Movies and TV: *One Flew Over the Cuckoo's Nest* became an iconic movie of the 1970s. Jack Nicholson's character, with his lovable rogue persona, is treated with ECT (electroconvulsive therapy — basically electric shocks). At the end of the movie a frontal lobotomy is aggressively forced upon him. Both these treatments are performed for the purposes of behaviour modification.
- Historical references: I like to tell the true story about the prominent attorney from Vermont in the USA who was treated for depression by

having his head held in a bucket of water. He drowned before they successfully treated the depression. Yes, it is a true story, but people forget to mention that it happened in 1806 — more than two hundred years ago. There is also a tendency to forget that orthodox medicine was in its infancy at this time, with leeches and bloodletting being other popular treatments, and no concept of germ theory and that fresh dressings were necessary for infected wounds.

- Churches: The Church of Scientology has spent considerable time and resources defaming psychiatry. Here's an example: an article entitled 'Psychiatry Causes Brain Damage', including helpful descriptions of ECT as the 'application of hog-slaughtering skills to humans, creating one of the most brutal techniques'. I have similar sentiments about the use of brainwashing on humans!

It is apparent that as long as these perceptions endure, millions of people worldwide are going without treatment. But the fear and ignorance that surround psychiatry are based in outdated images of this clinical practice. Psychiatry is a recognised school of medicine and has come a long way since those early horror stories in popular culture.

Oh no! I'm not that bad, am I?
— A quote from many, many clients

This quote illustrates one of the primary reasons for the negative view of all things psychiatric. Individuals believe that this is the absolute end of the road — that they are going 'stark raving' mad. They will soon be taken away in a straightjacket, locked up and the key thrown away.

In reality, depression is an illness like any other. The brain is just another organ, albeit a very specialised one that is central to everything we do and feel and say. Yet, internalising this factual information can be very difficult for some people, especially if they are unwell.

We readily accept that when something goes wrong with any of our other organs, we rest and we take medication. We do this often, without question. We make an effort to be 'kind' to that organ, limb or bone.

For instance, after a slight mishap on the ski slopes, you emerge looking a bit like this:

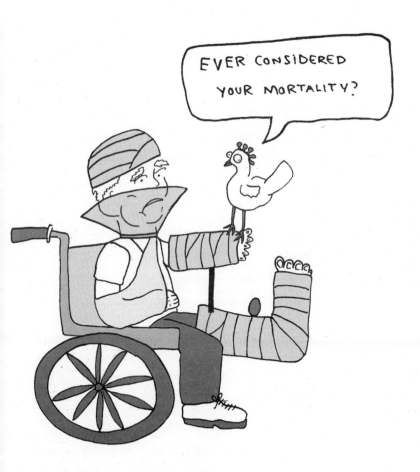

I'm going to take a punt and bet on the likelihood that you will not be entering a marathon any time soon. Instead, you will see a doctor and receive the medical treatment and rehabilitation support you need until you are recovered.

Yet, when the brain starts to exhibit symptoms of depression, such as poor concentration, attention and decision-making, you find yourself getting frustrated and annoyed with yourself. The first line of remedies is to work harder, drink more coffee and not ask for help — all the while expecting yourself to 'just get over it!'

The brain is just another — albeit the most important — organ of our body.

If your brain needs a break and some looking after for a while, *it doesn't mean you are a failure and it doesn't suggest a flaw in your personality.*

The stigma attached to mental illness (including depression and anxiety) certainly does come from films, media and society. However, it is usually your

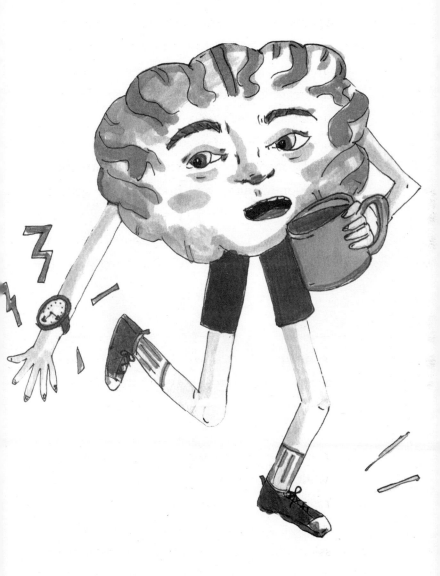

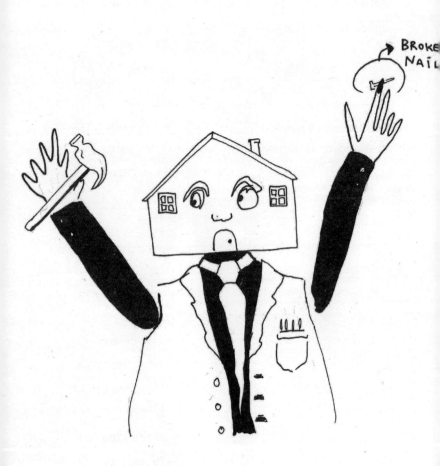

own internal sense of stigma that places the biggest roadblock in the way of treatment — your own fear and sense of failure.

WE LIVE IN OUR HEAD

Because our eyes, ears and breathing apparatus are attached to our head, and we think by using our brain, which is inside our head, it's not surprising that we sometimes feel as though we are living in our head.

As a result of this, there is a tendency to credit the brain with all sorts of mystical powers — the soul lives there, and perhaps the spirit lives there? Does it contain the ticket to the afterlife?

These beliefs lead to an overprotectiveness of the brain. A feeling that it's the organ that must never be medicated. That psychiatric interventions could result in irreparable damage to the 'self'.

This often goes hand-in-hand with the idea that psychiatrists are 'head-shrinkers' — the next closest thing to a witch doctor.

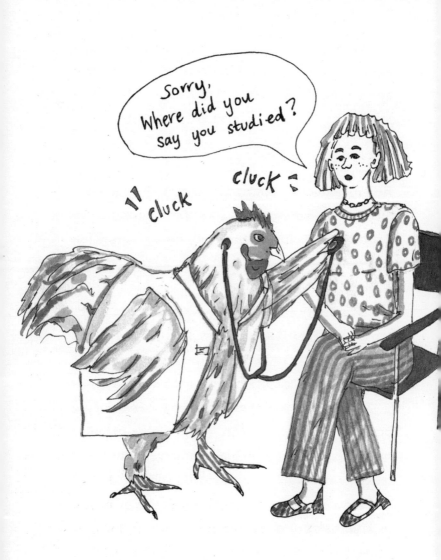

When the reality is:

Psychiatrists are doctors too.

You may still be a bit confused about the difference between psychologists and psychiatrists. The following information will help you differentiate. This is important, as it will assist you in deciding which direction to go in for help. (Your GP may also be able to help you with this.)

The primary role of the psychiatrist is the medical diagnosis and treatment of psychiatric ill health. Their particular, though not exclusive, emphasis is on biological treatments. (As discussed below, a psychologist cannot prescribe medication. But both professions engage in therapy.)

Certainly your GP can be of help, but they do not have specialist training in the area of mental health. The other big factor is that your doctor — as a result of 'pharma-economics' — only has access to certain antidepressants, usually those which are government-subsidised.

Don't get me wrong: the majority of people who present to their GP are treated successfully. The point I am making here is that psychiatrists are the medical specialists in mental health, just as oncologists are the medical specialists in the treatment of cancer.

The purpose of an initial meeting with a psychiatrist — as well as being a forum for gathering relevant information about the patient — is an evaluation. This process is to determine whether someone has a biochemical depression or one that is psychologically/environmentally based. A skilled psychiatrist should be able to differentiate between the two and make an informed prediction about the helpfulness of biological treatments (for example, medication or ECT), psychological therapies or a combination of both.

(I say 'skilled psychiatrist' because old-school psychiatry was very medically oriented. Back then psychological approaches — and psychologists — were considered a lowly adjunct among their professional colleagues. Clearly this is no longer the case, so you want to be in front of a psychiatrist who works within an integrated realm of mental health practitioners. If this is not apparent, don't be shy to ask — and find someone else if you need to!)

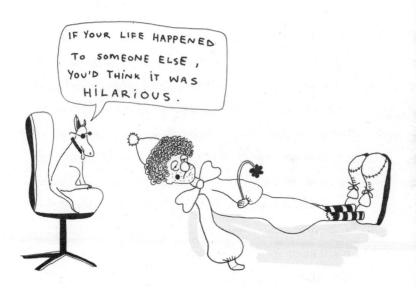

While on this topic, I also can't emphasise strongly enough that when you are deciding on who you should choose as your mental health professional (that is, if you have a choice), you need to make sure the 'fit' is right. In our academic literature we call this the 'interactive fit'.

Let me put it this way: you're up for a bit of retail therapy, so into the shoe shop you go. You know the style you want, you know the look you want, and also the outcome when you are out and about with the shoes on and living your best life. But much to your horror as you walk down the street, you find your new shoes don't fit — they're too tight, too rigid and too inflexible. You realise that you have spent all that money and there is no fit.

Therapists are no different. If the fit isn't right, don't buy more sessions week after week. If you tell a therapist or a psychiatrist this will be your last appointment, even if it is the first one, it is their problem if they take offence, not yours.

Shop until the fit is right.

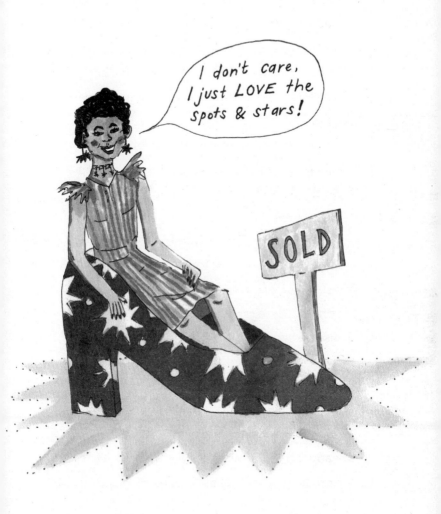

CHAPTER FIVE

TO BE MEDICATED OR NOT TO BE MEDICATED?

There is still a very powerful, almost omnipresent anti-medication lobby in today's world. And I would like to point out that this is far more prevalent with regard to psychiatric (psychotropic) medications than those used in other medical fields. Sure, some of you refuse to take antibiotics or anti-inflammatories — however, I suspect it's not that many of you.

Yet so many people I see are adamant that they do not need medication and they refuse to take psychotropics. How come? Well, here's a clue.

I have no idea how old you are, but I speculate with some certainty that some of you reading this were born in the 1960s or '70s, or your parents or grandparents were. Either way, you probably have either a personal experience or a cross-generational memory of not-so-good psychiatric treatment stories.

In the Western world, the 1960s was a time of significant social change. Nuclear families were still ensconced as a core social construct. Men would go out to work every day, leaving their wives and families at home, often in some tacky suburban box. Bored, depressed and anxious, the '60s housewives turned to their doctors for help.

The Rolling Stones acknowledged the dawning of the Age of Anxiety with their song 'Mother's Little Helper', about suburban housewives popping little yellow pills so they could cope with their husbands and kids.

Tranquillisers like benzodiazepines (note: *not* antidepressants) infiltrated our society under the guise of a harmless pharmacological panacea. They were sold to doctors as being free of side effects and non-addictive — a bit like Oxycodone in the 1990s. Worldwide, millions of people (mostly women) were prescribed these contemporary cure-alls. Problems started to occur, however, when people thought it was time to stop taking them.

It was then that scientists and practitioners realised the enormity of this 'medical blunder'. In defence of doctors — who were accused of being slaves to the drug companies, ready to prescribe the latest medication for a set of new golf clubs or a week in a tropical resort — it was about the times.

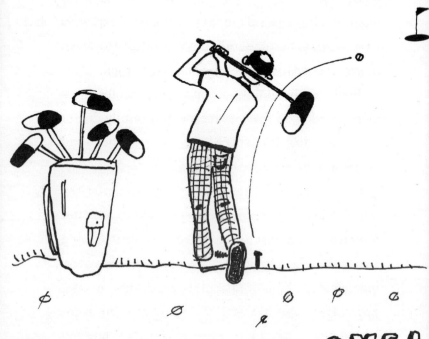

PARACETAM'OLE IN ONE!

In those days, pharmaceutical companies were able to spend excessively in their courtship of medical practitioners. I must admit to having flown business class around the South Pacific, all expenses paid, to speak at some conference or other. However, these practices are no longer allowed or legal.

Back to the point, despite these professional 'perks' — do you really perceive your family doctor to be a heartless drug pusher? That, rather than being interested in helping you, they are keen to get you addicted to prescription drugs to make a quick buck? — in the majority of cases it was not a matter of intentional malpractice. Don't think I am condoning the over-prescribing of anti-anxiety medications, but what I am suggesting is that doctors kept prescribing them and people continued taking them *because they worked* — they relieved anxiety. The problem was that they were also highly addictive.

Even though we are living in a different age now, people still have their memories of earlier times. And, as a result of this monumental f@#k-up, psychiatric pharmacological treatments are still considered to be the last rather than the first option.

THE NEW DRUG SCIENCE

I have to be honest with you: I once attended a conference at which a renowned psychiatrist put out this challenge to an audience of neuroscientists:

Can anyone here tell me exactly how anti-depressants work?
— Graham D. Burrows MD, Professor of Psychiatry, University of Melbourne, 2000

As I recall, there were no responses. The contemporary understanding, as far as I know, is that we fire a chemical into the dartboard of neurotransmitters, and we watch it work. The important part of this analogy is that *they do work*.

I have learned this from my own experience. I never really believed that medication was going to relieve the despair of my depression. However, I was desperate and, as I said earlier, my psychiatrist had already given me some leeway to try alternative approaches. Nothing helped in the slightest.

I asked my psychiatrist this question: 'Isn't it true that in many instances depressive illness will naturally pass?'

She replied: 'Yes, after a period of time — say, six to twelve months — and living in a world with no stress or strain.'

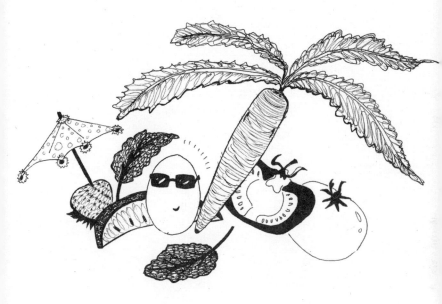

Mmm . . . fat chance, I thought to myself. Think I'll go for the medication.

Sure enough, after about three weeks on the medication, I started to feel little bits of my old 'self' return. I could write spontaneously, was able to begin conversations and even feel the return of a smile — an old, sorely missed companion.

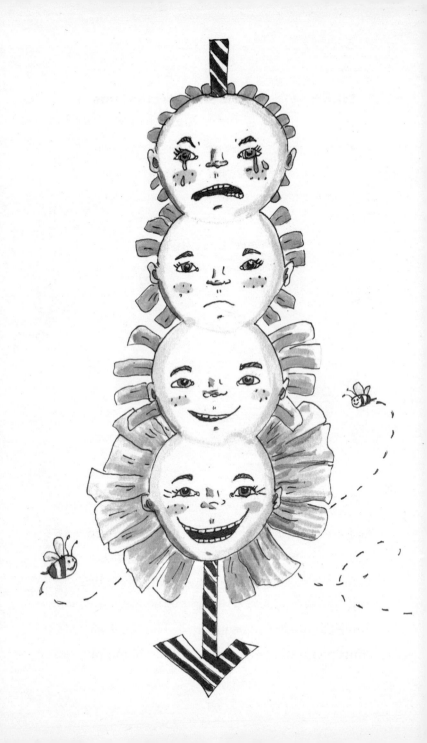

Stuff to know about antidepressants

- Antidepressants are not drugs of addiction or dependence, in that you don't require increasing doses to attain the same relief.
- When you stop taking them, there can be withdrawal effects with some — not all — antidepressants. Whether or not the product you are being prescribed has these properties, I strongly advise that this is monitored by your doctor or treating psychiatrist.
- There is no set amount of time to be on them. This is tailored for the individual and often correlates to the severity of the depression.

TYPES OF ANTIDEPRESSANTS

As I mentioned earlier, science has developed with regard to antidepressant medications.

Some antidepressant medications have been in use for over thirty years, such as monoamine oxidase inhibitors (MAOIs) and tricyclics: for example, amitriptyline, nortriptyline and clomipramine.

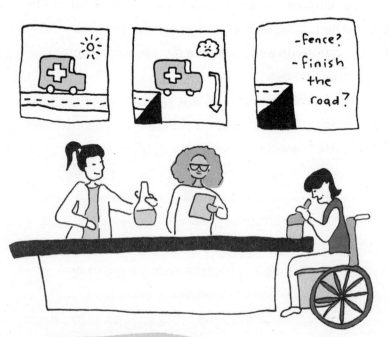

SCIENTISTS RESEARCH THE AMBULANCE AND THE HILL PROBLEM.

These were effective drugs, but the side effects were a real drag. To be on a therapeutic dose often meant taking as much as 75-100 mg a day. Apart from anything else, this dosing was guaranteed to blur your vision and give you a mouth like the bottom of a budgie cage.

However, although this generation of medications has been replaced, I have a soft spot for the use of some of them.

- I often recommend nortriptyline for worry and insomnia, but in low doses of around 10-25 mg daily (I call it a homoeopathic dose).
- Amitriptyline still holds a firm place in the chronic pain management field.
- Clomipramine is still a gold-card member for the treatment of obsessive compulsive disorder (OCD).

Tricyclics can often be used to 'augment' the newer drugs, to give them a bit more of a kick — just like mixing a cocktail.

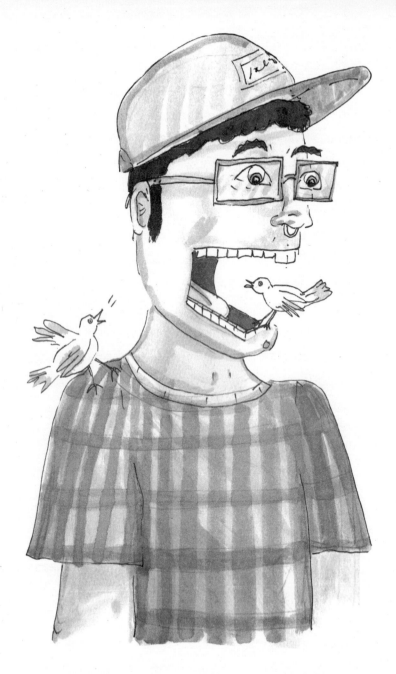

A mouth like the bottom of a budgie cage is a common side effect of some of the older antidepressant medications.

The new kids on the block

With these drugs having such unpleasant side effects, the race was on to create the next generation of antidepressants. In 1988 the leader of the pack was Prozac — the first SSRI (selective serotonin reuptake inhibitor) to be approved by the United States' Food and Drug Administration (FDA). Following closely were the sibling drugs such as Zoloft, Cipramil, Paxil and Aurorix. Each manufacturer offers different strengths and benefits in their brand, but these drugs have been found to be as effective as the tricyclics.

They were not without their side effects, either: I always laugh when I remember going to the launch of Aurorix (moclobemide), when the manufacturers proudly announced that their — and only their — medication did not have sexual dysfunction as a side effect.

Prozac also had its teething problems. It appeared as though Prozac had been tailored for the more melancholic-type depression I discussed earlier. However, its kick-start properties, intended to awaken the more vegetative depressive, overstimulated the anxious depressive, leading to increased cases of suicidality.

I remember asking my psychiatrist, Margaret, why I couldn't have Prozac, as it was such a fashion statement at the time. She replied, 'Because we can't take the risk of you going high again.' And that was the end of that.

What was next?

With the increasing awareness of the inextricable link between anxiety and depression, the hunt was on to find the pharmacological solution to this quandary. It arrived in the form of the SNRIs (serotonin-noradrenaline reuptake inhibitors), such as Pristiq, Effexor, Cymbalta and others. These worked on both serotonin and the adrenaline associated with anxiety.

Both the SSRIs and the SNRIs continue to be developed. Certainly, as we learn more about the relationship between anxiety and depression, these newer drugs will play an ever-increasing role in treatment of these conditions.

As you can see, there is a wide range of antidepressants available these days. Hence I reiterate the importance of considering a visit to a psychiatrist if the initial prescription from your GP offers minimal or no relief.

WHAT IF THE DRUGS DON'T WORK?

Yes, there is a small percentage of individuals who experience what we call a treatment refractory depression. This means that a number of anti-depressants have not worked, and nor have they worked in combination with psychological therapies. Fortunately this doesn't happen with a large number of people.

So what comes next with regard to biological treatments?

Transcranial magnetic stimulation (TMS)

This is described as a non-invasive procedure that uses magnetic fields to stimulate nerve cells in the brain, to improve symptoms of depression. I don't know a great deal about this technology, and won't pretend to, but success rates internationally are impressive. And what I can report is that while working in a clinic with a TMS system, I have seen a number of my treatment refractory patients benefit a great deal.

Some, but not all, need the odd top-up session. If you do arrive at this juncture the treating clinician will provide you with all the information you need to understand the technology of this exciting new adjunct to the treatment of depression.

Electroconvulsive therapy (ECT)

This first came into use in the medical arena in the late 1930s. As I mentioned earlier, because of the misuse, overuse and abuse of ECT, it not only fell out of favour as a treatment but also was actively lobbied against.

ECT consists of a split-second shock of between 75 and 150 volts of electricity. This is considered to be a small and safe current. It is administered in an attempt to induce a seizure, and it is the seizure that is thought to be responsible for the lifting of the mood.

Over the years I have worked with patients who have ECT as their treatment of choice. It works for them quickly, and they don't have to wait, suffering for months, to see if a medication is going to work.

When the TMS machine arrived at work, I asked my colleague: 'What is the difference between this treatment and ECT?' He replied, 'Similar approach, far less intrusive.'

Microdosing

Some of you may have heard of the practice of 'microdosing' substances such as LSD, ketamine and psilocybin to treat depression. I'm going to leave you to research those; they are gaining ground but experimentation is in the early stages of development.

My final word on this . . .

If I had not responded as well as I did to medication, would I have tried TMS? Yes, definitely.

If that didn't work, would I try ECT? Yes, particularly if it was recommended by my psychiatrist. These things are a matter of personal choice, and for some people ECT gives great results.

CHAPTER SIX

WHOSE COUCH IS IT ANYWAY — WHICH THERAPY IS FOR ME?

So now it's time to move away from the biological treatments and look at the contribution of psychological interventions. What we have established so far is that psychiatrists are medical experts who treat depression with biologically based interventions. At the risk of creating confusion, I should also mention that psychiatrists can be psychoanalysts and/or psychotherapists at the same time, and may offer some form of psychotherapeutic support.

This varies from country to country. Many American psychiatrists were educated in the field of psychoanalysis, but I don't think this is in vogue anymore. This has a lot to do with the advent of evidence-based cognitive behavioural therapy (CBT), which was far more appealing to insurance companies who had been forking out for the cost of analysis, which could have been three to five sessions per week for three to five years — with no guaranteed outcome!

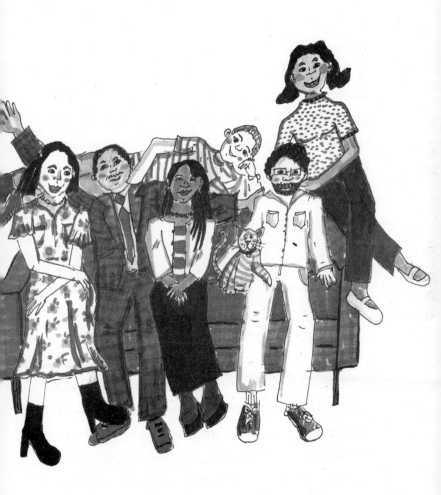

To summarise, a therapist can be a psychologist, a psychotherapist or a psychiatrist, who may have trained in psychoanalysis. But the main point is that psychotherapists, counsellors and psychologists are unable to prescribe medication.

So if you have a mental image of visiting the 'shrink', lying on the couch and being analysed, you're not completely wrong. But your analyst may not be a psychiatrist, and your psychiatrist or psychologist may not have a couch. Let's hope that's as clear as mud and move on . . .

SO WHICH THERAPY?

There are a number of different psychological therapies available. In my opinion, for depression, the greatest contribution is made by psychological therapies in conjunction with medication. In fact, there are certain CBT-based clinics in America where clinicians will not work with depressed patients unless they are medicated.

As I mentioned earlier, I will work with clients who aren't taking medication, depending on where the severity of their depression lies on the spectrum.

But when their score crosses the line into severe, I will insist on exploring medication, with only the odd exception.

I am a very eclectic clinician — because I've been a therapist for a very long time and have seen many approaches come and go. There are a lot of fads in my industry!

Here are a few statistics that you might find interesting: the global personal development industry was valued at US$38.28 billion in 2019, with a growth expectation of 5 per cent per year, providing a projected figure of US$56.66 billion by 2027. Old mate Tony Robbins clocks in at a mere US$480 million a year, with Deepak Chopra sitting on a modest US$150 million. Each to their own, I say.

I'm not mocking success — I mean, let's face it, I've been known to write the odd self-help book myself! I'm merely highlighting for you the enormity of the industry, the phenomenal diversity of the many, *many* treatment modalities, and the overwhelming amount of choice. I am a great believer in tailoring my approach to fit the individual I am working with and utilising what works for them.

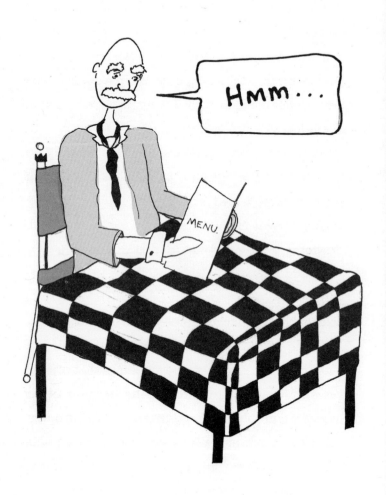

There can be such a thing as too much choice. It can be confusing and overwhelming.

When I am trying to find my way through a maze of seemingly infinite choices I will often turn to Wikipedia. In its researched list of available psychotherapies, I counted 87 *different types* of therapeutic approaches with the aim of improving mental health.

I forgot to mention that those 87 were only between the letters A–H! If I listed them all for you it would be an absolute maze of psychotherapeutic possibilities.

Which one? Which is the best? Which is perhaps the most fashionable? Which one will I like? Which one will my partner like?

To provide an answer to all of the above, let me introduce you to the common factors theory. This research proposes that despite the many types of interventions and techniques, there are common factors that account for much of the effectiveness of any psychological treatment.

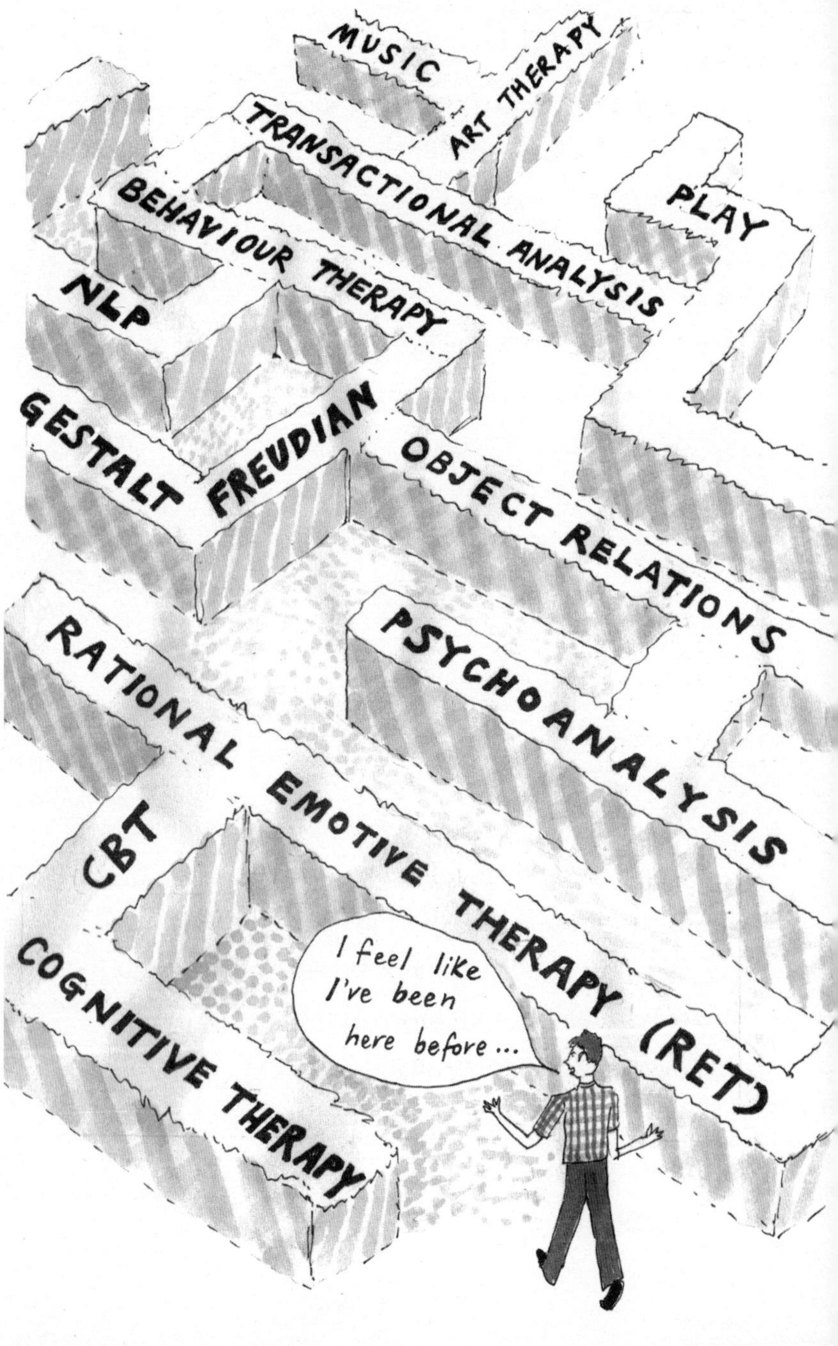
MUSIC
ART THERAPY
TRANSACTIONAL ANALYSIS
PLAY
BEHAVIOUR THERAPY
NLP
GESTALT
FREUDIAN
OBJECT RELATIONS
PSYCHOANALYSIS
RATIONAL EMOTIVE THERAPY (RET)
CBT
COGNITIVE THERAPY
I feel like I've been here before...

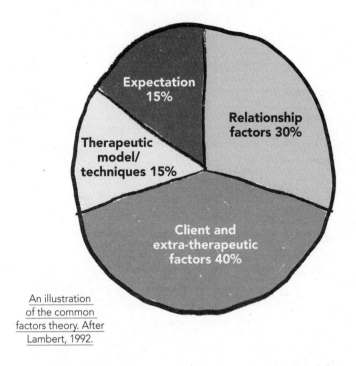

An illustration of the common factors theory. After Lambert, 1992.

As you can see in the pie chart, only 15 per cent of a successful outcome has to do with the therapeutic model or techniques used. Relationship factors, coming in at 30 per cent, include:

- empathy of the therapist
- goal consensus and collaboration
- positive regard and affirmation
- mastery of the therapist
- congruence/genuineness of both parties.

The point is that your relationship with the clinician is more important than the choice of technique.

Meta-study research indicates that the most recommended therapies for depression are:

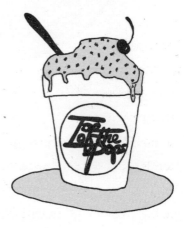

- cognitive therapy
- behavioural therapy
- cognitive behavioural therapy (see next page)
- dialectical behaviour therapy
- psychodynamic therapy
- interpersonal therapy.

But don't forget, in cases of more severe depression, these psychological therapies are most effective in conjunction with medication.

CBT is well known to many people, and certainly has a very impressive success rate in the treatment of depression and anxiety. It's the main modality I have integrated into my clinical practice. Yet many people who make an appointment will say to me:

I hope you don't do CBT. I've tried it and it doesn't work for me.

In my opinion, in these cases it was the relationship between the client and the therapist that didn't gel, not the therapy. So ask people you trust — your friends, your doctor — who they would recommend. Don't let the fear of stigma around depression hold you back from talking with others.

I hope this overview helps you understand a bit more about making a choice between different types of therapies. And if the therapy isn't working after six sessions, it's not going to. Go somewhere else. I mean, how many times would you go back to a hairdresser who messed up your hair?

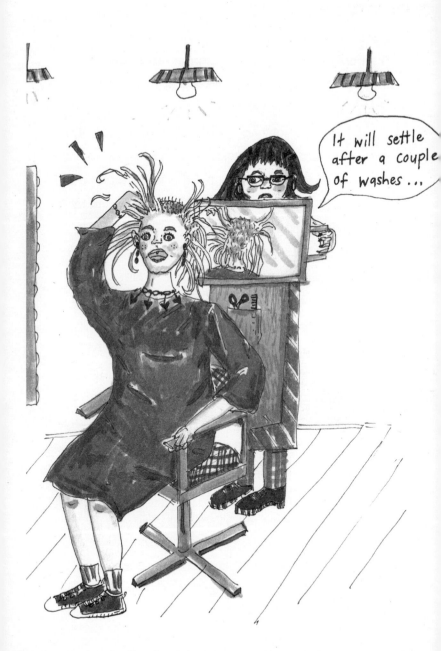

Would you keep going back to this hairdresser?

CHAPTER SEVEN

NATURAL THERAPIES — LOOKING BACK TO MOTHER NATURE

I carefully considered how to begin this discussion of what is now a very controversial topic within various schools of medicine. There are also significant discrepancies between nations, with many, such as Canada, the UK and parts of Europe, now developing and implementing the use of 'complementary alternative medicine' (CAM).

HISTORICALLY . . .

Our relationship with the use of medicinal plants is dated by archaeological evidence back to the Palaeolithic age, approximately 60,000 years ago. The first written record of it was created on clay tablets over 5000 years ago by the Sumerians in ancient Mesopotamia. So healing with plants is as old as humanity itself. And let's not forget that nations such as China and India have a 6000-year history with plant, herbal and other natural therapies.

As one of my favourite geniuses once said:

Look deep into nature, and then you will understand everything better.
— Albert Einstein

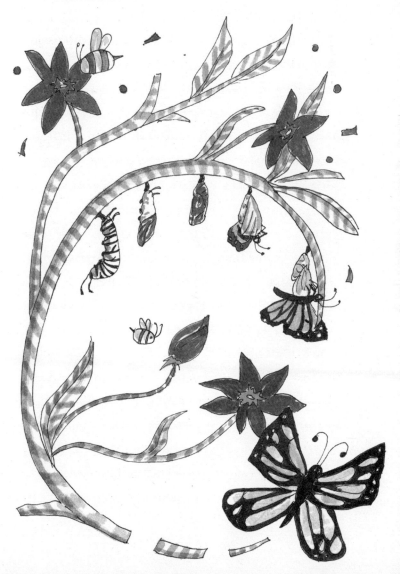

During the early modern period — from the late 1400s to the 1700s — university-trained physicians were scarce and people would often turn to 'wise women' for herbal healing. However, the bad news was that if things didn't work out too well, the wise women were accused of witchcraft. Even more bad news: during this early modern era it has been estimated that tens of thousands of people were executed or burned at the stake for 'witchcraft'. No wonder the practice became unfashionable! Particularly if you were a woman during the rise of patriarchal governing systems.

The early part of the nineteenth century was a turning point with regard to knowledge about and the use of medicinal plants: the poppy, quinine (made from bark), pomegranate. The development of chemical methods found other active substances in medicinal plants, such as tannins, vitamins and hormones.

Modern Western medicine, as we now know it, started to emerge after the Industrial Revolution in the eighteenth century. There was enormous economic, industrial and population growth, accompanied by an increasing number of people travelling across continents and oceans.

Scientists began to understand how bacteria and viruses worked. At the same time, much of the reduction in mortality rates from the late nineteenth century had more to do with public health measures such as running water, sanitation, waste disposal and hand washing, and hence cannot necessarily be ascribed to Western pharmacology.

THE NEED FOR BULK, SPEED AND BIG PHARMA

Chemists and scientists continued to hunt for cures for the ever-increasing number of ailments and diseases in this modern era. For instance, in 1897 a group of German chemists produced the first form of aspirin using a synthetic version of salicin, which can be derived from willow bark. It was to become a global economic success.

We were now able to mimic the properties of medicinal plants via the use of synthetics. The seeds of the opium poppy were tweaked into heroin and morphine, and then came the development of methadone and our most recent horror show, Oxycodone and fentanyl.

At the time of writing I have just learned of the death of a wonderful and vibrant young man who was once a client of mine. Preparing for a decadent evening, he was planning on buzzing on a bit of cocaine when some devil turned up with cocaine cut with fentanyl, making it go further and hence putting more money in his pocket! Fentanyl is fifty to a hundred times more potent than morphine, and lethal in the smallest of doses. My former client took it and was instantly brain-dead, and was declared clinically dead an hour later. What a great tragedy, but he is just one of the many victims of the street world of synthetic opiates, which are far more deadly than Mother Nature's original pain relief, the good old poppy.

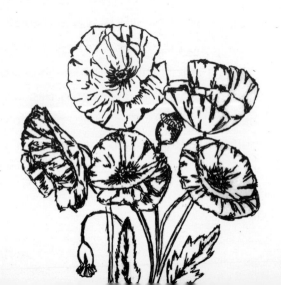

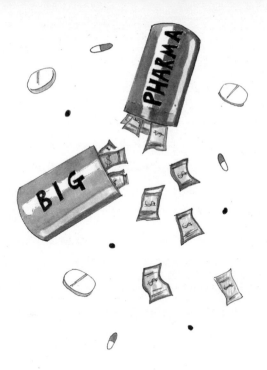

As the global demand for pharmaceuticals continued to expand in the twentieth century, so did the wealth and power of 'Big Pharma', the manufacturers of these drugs — along with the politics and the 'profits above all' mentality.

However, if we look at the research into Covid and the number of lives saved by the rapid manufacture of vaccines by pharmaceutical companies, I encourage you to not be too cynical. Where would we be without antibiotics, penicillin and the polio vaccine, treatments for AIDS, depression, schizophrenia, bipolar and so on and so forth? It ain't all bad.

COMPLEMENTARY ALTERNATIVE
MEDICINES AND DEPRESSION

The science that I introduced earlier included research into drugs for mental illness. After that huge f@#k-up with the benzodiazepines (see page 111), it of course is far from surprising that many people wanted to return to all things natural, avoiding 'Big Pharma' and orthodox medications.

This trend can also be seen in the healthier diet, organics and anti-gluten movements. However, over-the-counter natural supplements are not without their own significant downsides and limitations within the field of mental health.

Here are the most common natural therapies for depression.

- **Omega-3 fatty acids**: still currently being studied as a possible treatment for depression, although they are considered generally safe to take.
- **Saffron**: may improve some symptoms of mild depression, but still needs more research.
- **5-HTP**: 5-Hydroxytryptophan, also known as oxitriptan, may play a role in improving levels of serotonin (a mood chemical). However, there

are safety concerns around uninformed dosing, in that it could contribute towards serotonin syndrome (an adverse reaction to an excess of serotonin). Evidence of its efficacy is still preliminary.

- **CBD oil**: cannabidiol, the active ingredient in cannabis, has taken the modern medical world by storm in certain countries, and is used for various conditions. There is increasing research that shows CBD has anti-stress effects, which may reduce depression related to stress. I am not averse to recommending my clients to a medically qualified 'green' doctor to give CBD a try, but primarily for anxiety disorders.

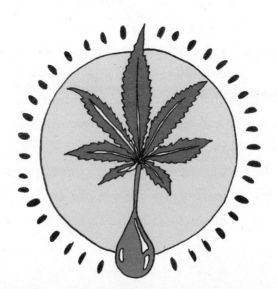

- **St John's wort**: appears to be helpful in the treatment of mild/moderate depressions — 'the blues'. However, it is known to interfere with other medications, including antidepressants, birth control and blood thinners.

Because these nutritional and dietary supplements do not need to go through the rigorous requirements of agencies such as the FDA, you can't always be certain of what you're buying. Hence my advice is to make sure you are buying from a reputable company, and discuss it with your healthcare provider.

Neither prescription medicines nor complementary alternative medicines (CAMs) can be guaranteed safe. People assume that natural medicines *must* be safe, because they are 'natural'. However, we are no longer talking about well-meaning 'wise women' picking herbs; we are talking about an industry that in 2021 was valued at US$100 billion, with a projected growth by 2028 to US$404.66 billion.

Where there is a trend and a need, there is a marketer, closely followed by a corporation out to make a profit.

MY TOP TIPS ON NATURAL THERAPIES

- Buy from a reputable company.
- Check with your healthcare provider before starting to take any natural remedy.
- Make sure you are seeing a naturopath, herbalist or functional medicine specialist, or a doctor with specialist training in these areas.
- These therapies for depression, at this stage, are showing to be helpful, but only for mild/moderate depression — 'the blues'. I would not recommend them for clinical depression, especially not as a primary treatment intervention.

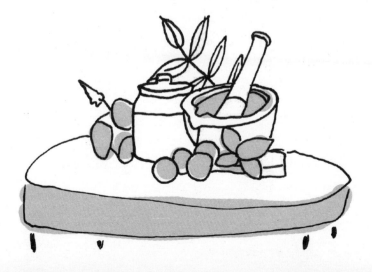

CHAPTER EIGHT

DEPRESSION — WHAT'S GOD GOT TO DO WITH IT?

S o far I have focused on health-based services: psychology, psychiatry, naturopathy and so on. Then it occurred to me that I have not yet acknowledged the relationship many people have with their church, their chosen spiritual beliefs and/or their spirituality as it relates to their culture, which can play an important part in their experience of and treatment for depression.

Out of the world population of 7.3 billion in 2018, 2.3 billion (31.2 per cent) believed in the Christian God, with the Muslim faith accounting for 1.8 billion (24.1 per cent), Hindus 1.1 billion (15.1 per cent) and Buddhists 500 million (6.9 per cent). That's a lot of people! In 2021 it was estimated that about 85 per cent of the world's people identify with a religion.

Faith also appears to be growing amongst the younger population, who are seeking to affiliate with groups that believe in kindness, helping those in need and saving the planet.

Spirituality remains a very important dimension

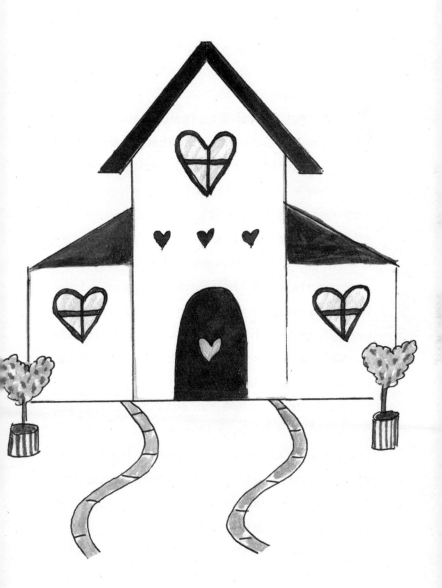

of people's lives, whether or not they practise orthodox religion. It is inherent, intrinsic, inseparable from who we are. Through our culture, our mythology and symbols, our memories and dreams, it is our ancestry.

It is not my goal to discuss the differences between the various religious denominations as they relate to the treatment of depression. However, as a healer, I do believe that it is important to acknowledge and work within the realm of an individual's faith and concept of spirituality.

It is also essential to incorporate the spiritual community within the support system for the depressed person and their family. With our struggling mental health systems worldwide, it is vital that additional support is resourced from elsewhere in the person's community.

This is not only to do with access to public health resources; it may be that the person you feel most comfortable talking to about your distress is your minister or spiritual counsellor. This in turn can often lead to advice to seek specialist medical help.

I personally have worked with clergy who have studied mental health and psychological therapies.

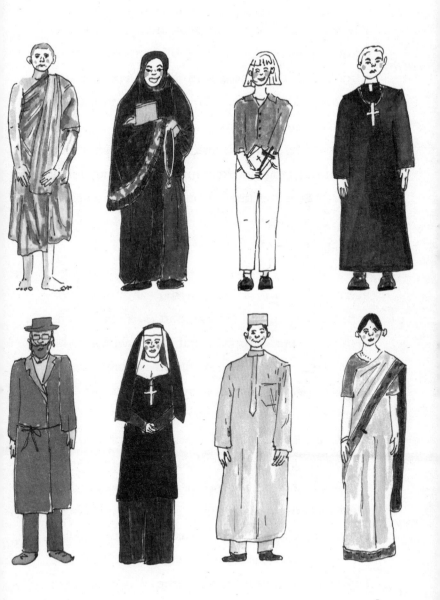

The way I see it is that if practitioners are serious about a 'holistic' approach, they need to be accommodating and respectful of other forms of help.

Healing comes from co-operation, not from elitism, competition and ownership of the cure.

It is important that you can assertively express your needs and your loved one's wishes in this complex sphere of spirituality. Within the 'holistic' approach to the treatment of mood instability — whether it be the blues or clinical depression — it is important to acknowledge both the contributions and limitations of spiritual counsel of any denomination.

I find this to be particularly important within those cultures who do not believe in the existence of mental illness, and hence may be opposed to Western orthodox medicine. I have found this in the work I have done in the Asia-Pacific region. For example, I was once invited to speak to a group of Japanese psychiatric clinicians at a neuroscience summit. They spoke of the difficulties they were having trying to convince their patients to accept depression as an illness, and battling against the belief in 'losing face'.

I suggested to them that they emphasise the fact that the brain is an organ of the body and, just like any other organ, if it is strained and not functioning, the approach is parallel to the treatment of any other organ. I have no idea how they got on. It is exceptionally hard work trying to break through ingrained cultural belief systems.

THE PLACE OF FAITH

It is my experience that people with depression can appear, within a spiritual framework, to be undergoing a crisis of faith, when in fact the crisis of being (existential crisis) is actually depression, and with the right treatment the faith will return undisturbed.

Therefore, depression may appear as a crisis of faith, but it is more than that: it is an illness, and it is vital to the individual's wellbeing to differentiate between the two.

Wise words from a wise man

Many years ago I spoke with an Anglican minister named Jeremy who was also trained in psychotherapy. His thoughts and observations were as follows:

Certainly there is a nervousness among the clergy with regard to psychiatry and drug therapy. Just as I know that among a lot of psychotherapists and psychiatrists there is a total dismissal of the spiritual-helping professions. It is as if they are dismissed as being well-meaning amateurs with no status.

We need to work together. It's not as simple as the acupuncturist who will take away your disease, the confessor who will take away your guilt, and the cure-all faith healer.

In the treatment of depression, spiritual guidance is only one component of the overall 'healing package'.

A faith metaphor

This little anecdote was sent to me by a wonderful man who is a psychiatrist and a man of faith:

A woman of great faith lived in a home that was threatened by flood. When the government sent a radio message to everyone that they should escape to higher ground, she stayed where she was. 'God will save me,' she told her neighbours.

The floodwaters rose so high that they flooded the ground floor of her house and she had to relocate upstairs. The local civil defence people rowed up to her upstairs window in a boat to try to rescue her, but she refused. 'God will save me,' she told them.

The flood got even worse and she ended up clinging to the TV antenna on her roof. The air force sent a helicopter. They lowered a ladder for her to climb up but she stayed where she was, shouting up to the rescue workers: 'Don't worry, God will save me!'

*Then the floodwaters rose even higher, swept
her away, and she drowned. When she
reached heaven, she was very confused and
asked an angel to explain why God hadn't
saved her. The angel was surprised. 'Oh my
dear, we sent you a radio message, then a
boat, and finally a helicopter, just for you.
What on earth were you waiting for?'*

I often share this sentiment with my religious
clients, by suggesting to them that perhaps
antidepressant medications and psychotherapy are
further examples of divine intervention; that the
'gift' to be able to heal via medicine and technology
is a skill we have been provided with, like the radio
message, the boat and the helicopter. This is just
one of many interpretations of the world we live in!

Some more wise words

*The religion of the future will be a cosmic
religion. It will have to transcend a personal
God and avoid dogma and theology. Encom-
passing both the natural and the spiritual.*

It will have to be based on a religious sense arising from the experience of all things, natural and spiritual, considered as a meaningful unity.

— Author unknown

Sometimes these words are attributed to Albert Einstein but, whether it was him or not, whoever wrote them was on to something.

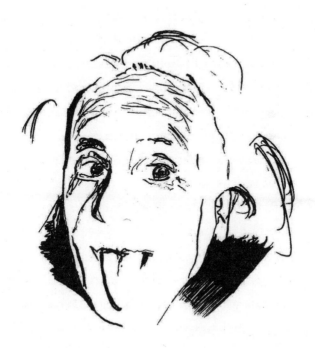

MY TOP TIPS FOR PEOPLE OF FAITH

- Request that your spirituality/cultural beliefs be acknowledged when dealing with health professionals.

- You may choose to deal with your anguish through a spiritual outlet, seeking out the support of your church and the community. But hoping that if only you or your loved one would regain their faith the depression would go away is not practical, as it is unlikely to happen.

- If you or your loved one are looking for a cure by means of faith healing, I recommend the reading of evidence-based educational material.

- Scientific research has proved the 'healing power of prayer'. Hence this can be helpful and contribute to psychological wellness, in the same way as meditation and mindfulness.

- Your spiritual counsellor or minister is not traditionally trained in psychotherapy or psychiatric diagnosis. However, they can be of great support at this time, and may also be able to guide you in the right direction if you don't know which way to turn.

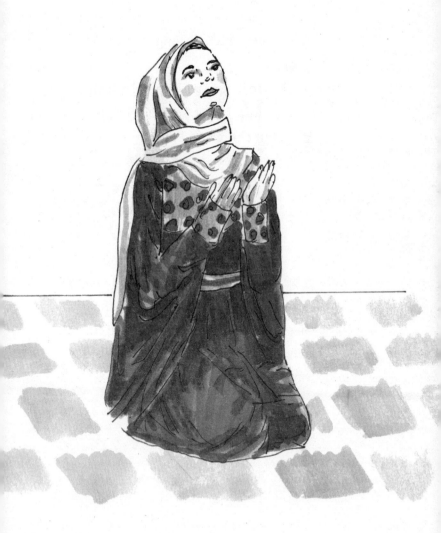

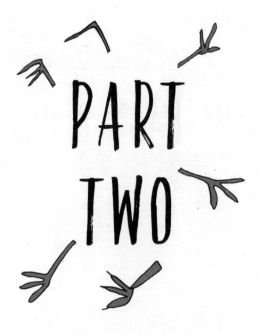

PART
TWO

CHAPTER NINE

THE BABY BLUES AND BEYOND

B aby blues are feelings of sadness that you may experience after having a baby. Up to 80 per cent of new parents — and not just the person who has given birth — experience the baby blues. It can affect new parents of any race, age, income, culture or education level.

The key difference between the baby blues and postnatal depression is the severity of the symptoms. These do differ between women, as do the number of symptoms experienced.

Medical intervention is not required unless the symptoms hang around for longer than a few weeks. It is at this stage that the 'blues' may have morphed into depression, in which case treatment will need to be explored.

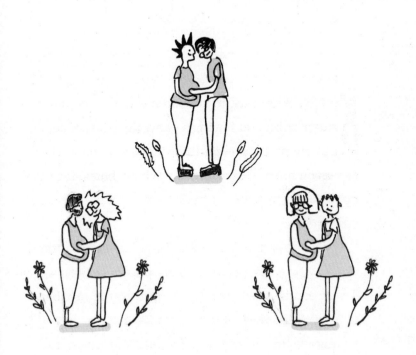

Important note: When it comes to the 'baby blues', and especially postnatal depression, it is important to remember that you are not at fault. What you are experiencing is *an illness and not a reflection of you as a mother or as a woman.*

SOME STATISTICS

Although it differs across countries, it is very common to experience the 'baby blues'. However, it is estimated that between 10 and 20 per cent of mothers are affected by the more serious condition postnatal depression, and in very rare instances the even more severe postpartum psychosis. The onset of postnatal depression occurs within six weeks of giving birth, although it can emerge for up to a year after the baby is born.

I have found in my practice that women often experience a severe drop in mood after stopping breastfeeding, which is not necessarily a sign that they are developing postnatal depression. It appears to be strongly correlated with the decrease and eventual cessation of nature's production of the hormone oxytocin. This hormone has gathered a reputation of being the 'love' or 'cuddle' hormone, as it is released when human beings snuggle up or bond socially.

When a mother breastfeeds, her body makes the hormones prolactin and oxytocin. Oxytocin produces a peaceful, nurturing feeling that allows her to relax and focus on the baby, and also

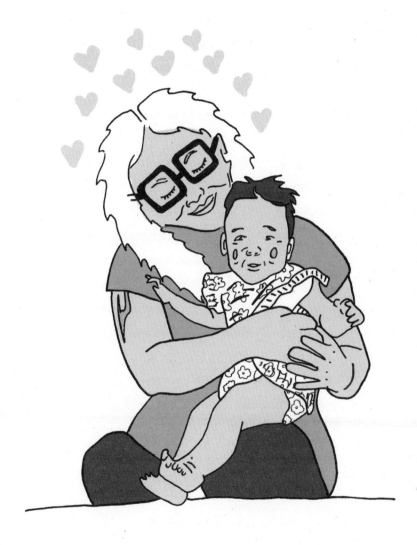

contributes to ease of milk release. It also promotes a strong sense of love and attachment between mother and baby. So when breastfeeding stops it can take a while for the mother's brain and body to readjust.

THE BABY BLUES

Baby blues are a common phenomenon, and although they do not require a lot of medical attention, they can still be very distressing. Albeit short-lived, they can be a highly unpleasant experience for new mothers. There is no one cause, and nor are some women more likely to suffer than others.

Symptoms include the following:

Physical symptoms

- not sleeping well, and feeling tired no matter how much sleep you've had
- lack of energy
- food cravings or loss of appetite.

Psychological/emotional symptoms

- feeling constantly anxious
- lacking confidence and feeling 'I'm not myself'
- overwhelming feelings of sadness
- feeling confused and nervous.

Reactions

- irritability with everyone
- feeling hurt easily and crying a lot
- lack of feeling for the baby.

These symptoms can pass quickly, and of course can be attributed to sleep deprivation, but research suggests a number of contributing factors can be at work. These include:

- hormonal changes
- the physical and mental stresses of labour
- the social changes involved in transitioning from being at work to being home in a more isolated position.

I would speculate that, as a new mother, you have been looking forward to your baby arriving. So to feel sad, anxious and lacking in confidence seems like a total contradiction, when you think of how you 'should' be feeling.

As I mentioned earlier, medical intervention is not required unless the symptoms hang around for longer than a few weeks. It is at this stage that the 'baby blues' may have morphed into depression, in which case treatment will need to be explored.

The most important thing that I can suggest is that you talk about what you are experiencing.

The benefits are twofold:

1. You establish a pathway to open communication with your loved ones, which acts as a preventative measure if things start to get worse and the blues develop into postnatal depression.
2. This openness enables you to ask for help. Ask not only for practical help, but also for a bit of assistance with the baby so that you can have a day spa or a good soak in a bath surrounded by beautiful aromatherapy candles. 'Don't ask, don't get.'

Remember, your loved ones don't necessarily know what you need. So I encourage you to be very open about your experience and don't be shy to ask for support. As I said earlier, this subjective experience is complicated and is not because you are a bad mother or a bad person.

Anyone involved with the new mother can offer support by listening to the mother's feelings and encouraging her to talk. Practical support, like a bit of housework, shopping or doing some washing, never goes amiss.

Don't forget to indulge her with the odd massage or beauty spa visit, or invite a couple of her friends around for a catch-up.

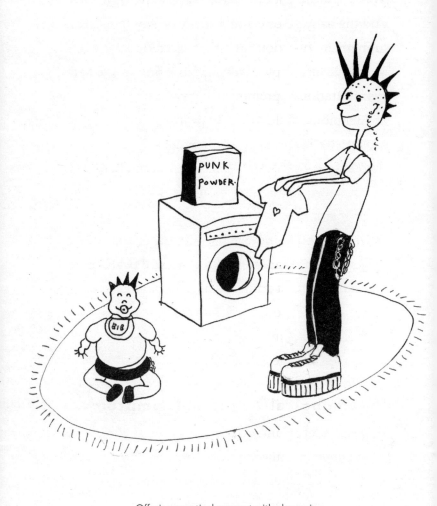

Offering practical support with chores is a
good way to help new parents.

POSTNATAL DEPRESSION

The key difference between postnatal depression and the baby blues is the severity of the symptoms, and their duration. This does differ between women. The symptoms can occur separately or be a manifestation of prolonged 'baby blues'.

Symptoms include the following:

Physical symptoms

- sleep disturbance, unable to get to sleep, waking early
- headaches
- general pains and feelings of being unwell (for example, chest pains, heart palpitations)
- hyperventilation, panic attacks
- loss of sexual interest
- marked change in appetite.

Psychological/emotional symptoms

- despondency and despair
- feeling inadequate, unable to cope
- a sense of hopelessness and powerlessness
- inability to concentrate, think clearly or remember things. I've had a few new mums say

to me: 'It's almost like my brain disappeared with the placenta.'

- thoughts of suicide, strange thoughts or fantasies
- lack of interest in activities once enjoyed (anhedonia)
- excessive concern over the baby's health.

Reactions

- extreme or unusual behaviour
- anxiety, along with new fears or phobias
- not wanting to go out or be with people
- nightmares
- feelings of being out of control or 'going crazy'
- no feelings for the baby, or anger towards the baby
- feelings of extreme guilt.

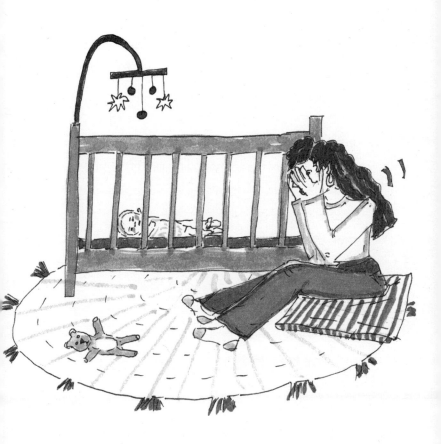

Important information

As the other parent or a loved one, you may notice and be concerned about the new mum displaying these symptoms, before she herself will acknowledge there is a problem. Think of the shame experienced by a new mother who feels nothing, and at times feels hostile towards her newborn. These are feelings she doesn't want to tell anybody about. She can often be afraid of appearing 'mentally ill', or not capable of looking after her child. As time progresses, under the cloud of depression, she begins to hate herself, she hates the baby and becomes convinced that you and everybody else around her hates her as well. Talking about this may not be easy. Hence, a lot of mothers will try to convince themselves and others that it is just the 'blues' and things will resolve any day — but they won't.

What causes postnatal depression

There are numerous contributing factors to postnatal depression, from hormonal issues to social problems. The following aspects are thought to increase the risk factor for women:

- stressful or unplanned pregnancy
- difficult childbirth
- isolation, lack of family support
- career change from paid employment and therefore loss of identity (especially for women over thirty)
- the recent death of a close friend or family member
- previous abortion, cot death, stillbirth or miscarriage
- unresolved issues from childhood / poor relationship with own mother
- increased workload at home, especially with a 'difficult' baby
- juggling a career and a new baby.

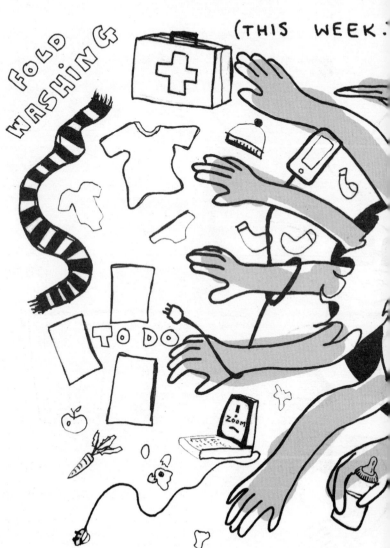

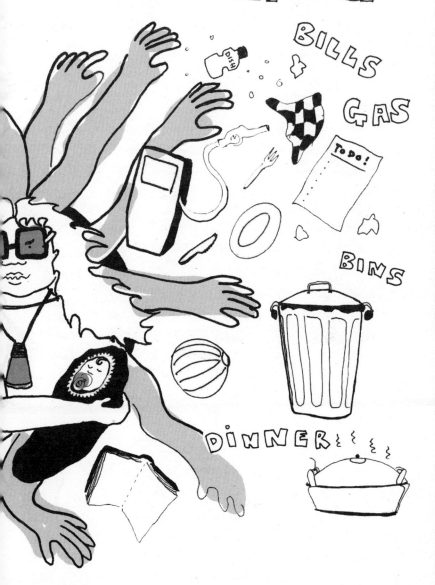

POSTNATAL PSYCHOSIS

This is a very rare form of maternal depression — with only one woman in 1000 estimated to suffer from this postnatal phenomenon.

Psychosis refers to a total loss of reality. It usually comes on in a very quick and spectacular manner within the first few weeks after giving birth, but the onset can be within hours of delivery. It can be extremely scary, especially if the new mother has never experienced psychosis before. It is additionally traumatic because it is difficult for the mother to differentiate between reality and the illness playing tricks on her brain.

Symptoms include the following:

Physical symptoms

- refusal to eat
- inability to stop being busy
- frantic, excessive energy
- loss of sexual interest.

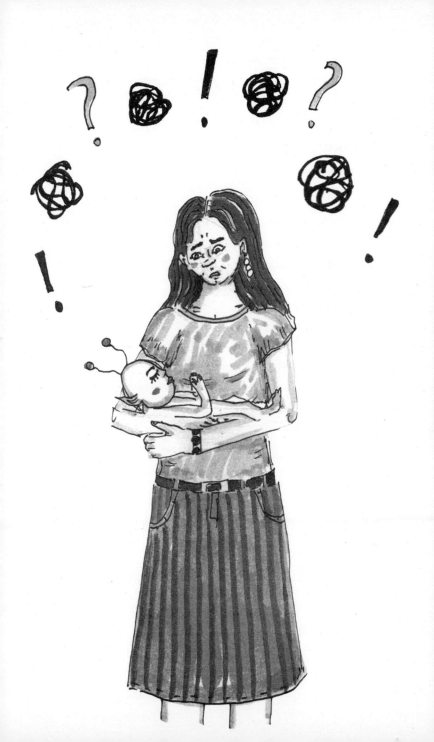

Psychological/emotional symptoms

- extreme confusion
- feelings of guilt and remorse
- loss of memory
- becoming incoherent
- thoughts of suicide
- bizarre hallucinations (usually auditory), delusions — belief in things that are not real
- thoughts of infanticide (killing the baby).

Reactions

- suspiciousness
- preoccupation with trivial matters
- irrational statements and reactions.

Once again, the causes are not fully understood, but the following are possibilities:

- a previous history of a similar disorder
- close relatives with similar disorders
- biochemical and/or psychological stress associated with childbirth.

Postnatal psychosis is a very serious condition, and medication and psychiatric care are essential. It tends to be an acute, often short-term illness, with 95 per cent of sufferers recovering well after treatment, but hospitalisation may be required for the safety of both mother and child.

With these more serious maternal depressions, interventions need to occur as quickly as possible, as these early weeks and months are so necessary for attachment and bonding. *Don't waste time before getting help.*

MEDICATION CONCERNS

Of course, no expectant mother wants to think about ingesting drugs during pregnancy and breast-feeding. Therefore deciding how to treat depression during pregnancy isn't easy.

The risks and benefits of taking medication

during pregnancy must be weighed up carefully. Work with your healthcare provider to make an informed choice that gives you — and your baby — the best chance for long-term health and wellbeing. Although antidepressants are considered low risk with regard to causing birth defects, the type and amount of medication needs to be carefully considered.

Particularly in the third trimester, when the baby is fully formed, the main concern of healthcare providers is the wellbeing of the mother. Pregnant mothers do commit suicide — not in large numbers, but the point is that if the mother is not well, the impact on the baby both before and after birth outweighs the impact of taking anti-depressant medications.

Although taking medication after the birth of the baby is not such a frightening thought, some new mothers still remain very reluctant. With postnatal psychosis, medication *is a must*. The longer the mother remains unwell and unable to connect with her baby, the more damage is done to that essential early bonding and attachment.

Research tells us that severe depression before,

during and after pregnancy can have lasting negative effects on new mothers and their young children. A mother's inability to care for and form an attachment with her baby can affect the child's long-term social, emotional, physical and cognitive development. Of course, this is true for any primary carer of the baby, whether they are the biological mother or not.

Maternal mental health specialists are the first port of call for advice; however, your psychiatrist and/or primary healthcare provider should be knowledgeable in this area or able to refer you to a specialist. Psychotherapy can again help treat mild/moderate depression.

PARENT NUMBER TWO
MATTERS TOO

We now live in a world where the orthodox structure of Mum, Dad and the kids may remain the norm, but we can also have two mums, two dads, one mum and a sperm donor, and transgender parents. Hence 'parent number two' becomes an even more important and at times complex consideration.

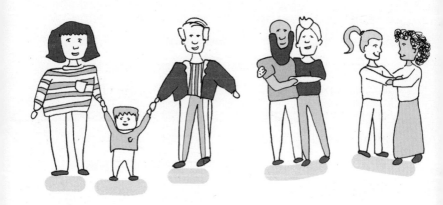

There can no longer be a reductionistic focus on the biological parent. Even if both parents are biological, this does not mean that the parent who gives birth is the primary parent; some biological mothers return to work and 'parent number two' becomes the stay-at-home primary parent.

So much research emphasis has been placed on the biological parent and their subsequent bonding with the baby, as if the blood connection was the ultimate relationship. If this was the case, then how does one explain the child abuse that can sometimes occur in biologically based relationships? A blood relationship does not necessarily guarantee the wellbeing of the infant.

Attachment theory

Primary caregivers who are available and responsive to an infant's needs allow the child to develop a sense of security. The infant learns that the caregiver is dependable, which creates a secure base for the child to then explore the world. This clarifies the fact that the parent who is there consistently and reliably is the child's primary attachment.

However, 'parent number two' can experience a lot of the same vulnerability and responsibility historically attached to the primary parent. Parent number two is exposed to the same amount of sleep deprivation and hence exhaustion, which contributes to mood dips.

It is also understood that parents with existing anxiety are more prone to postnatal depression, as the vulnerability that goes with being responsible for a newborn exacerbates anxiety and worry.

Also, if parent number two is the main financial provider, a whole other set of worries can occur. The child that you have dreamed of somehow morphs into a burden, placing additional strain on your emotional and physical wellbeing and taking you closer to the edge of a potential depressive response.

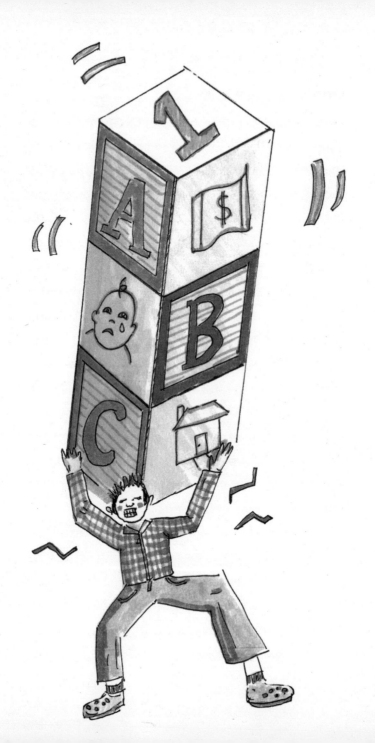

Don't forget me!

In my clinical experience, after the birth of the child the focus of the health professionals is on the biological mother. This is especially the case if there is a diagnosis of postnatal depression. Once the diagnosis has been made, the focus of the treatment is on the mother, too, as practitioners will be concerned with the infant's safety around her. Parent number two tends to be overlooked in this process — but they will also be going through a period of considerable stress and change.

As parent number two, you will have been faced with significant changes in your relationship, with the baby now being the main focus. You will have had very little time together, and intimacy has likely been replaced by fatigue and late-night feeds. It is not out of the ordinary if you feel very isolated during this time.

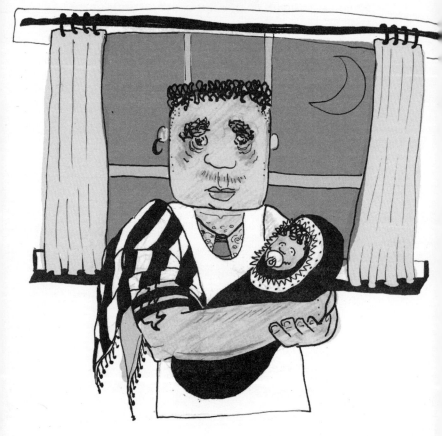

Story from a father

One of my clients shared this story with me.

When my wife Rachel began talking to me about her thoughts of harming our child, I contacted our family GP. A team of visiting nurses turned up, and I started to feel that they were insinuating that I was the problem, that I was the reason that she was feeling doubtful and tearful.

When Rachel was eventually hospitalised I did everything I could to keep the house running. I would have greatly appreciated somebody explaining to the family what was happening, so that extended family could understand and offer support.

When I reached out to the mental health professionals, there were times when I felt that the psychiatrist really hadn't explained things to me all that well, given that I was the main support person.

Being informed of what to expect would have been helpful. You need to know that it's not necessarily something you have done, or not done, it's just part of the deal with postnatal depression.

I guess the other thing I learned is that it is important to discuss things. The focus during antenatal classes is on the positive. I think there should be a lot more emphasis on the issues involved in having a child, and this education should include the strain on parent number two as well as the biological mother.

My top tips for the number twos

- There will be times when you feel despondent and alienated. Try not to take things personally, and make sure that you develop a support system for yourself.
- Don't be afraid to talk to others about how you are feeling — it helps, and also begins to destigmatise your experience, so you're not left feeling that you're a bad parent or partner.
- Be assertive with health professionals. Request

to be involved and kept informed of any changes in medications or major clinical decision-making with regard to the mother.

- Follow your instincts. If you feel that your partner is getting worse, or is coming off their medication too soon, express your concerns.
- In very severe cases, as with postnatal psychosis, it may be best for your partner to be hospitalised. **This does not mean you have failed.** It is a matter of what is best for her and the baby at this time.
- Your help is valuable in the most practical of ways — helping with chores around the house, cooking meals, bathing the baby, doing the shopping. Get her a bit of indulgence.
- Inform certain people at work about what is going on, so that you can perhaps leave work a little early or take time off when needed.
- Encourage your partner to talk about how she is feeling, and try not to be judgemental about unpleasant thoughts she may reveal. She will already be experiencing shame and self-criticism, and will withdraw if you react the same way.

- Keep visits from friends and family at a moderate level. Large social gatherings are not advisable — there will be plenty more time for this later, once she is well.
- Organise breaks for both of you — short walks, time away from the house.
- Get up to the baby at night and try to let your partner sleep through, minimising sleep disturbance.
- Don't forget to say 'I love you'.

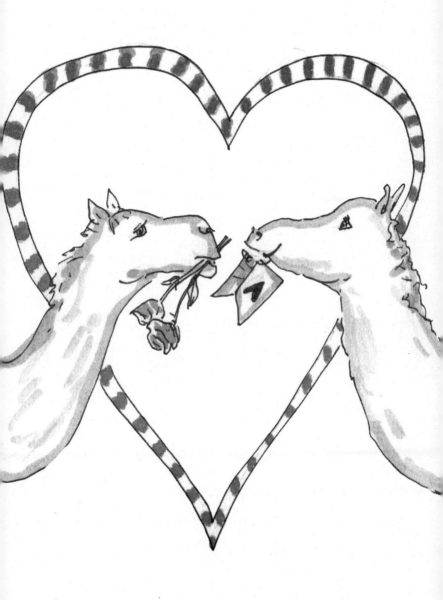

CHAPTER TEN

TEENAGE DEPRESSION — MORE THAN JUST A PHASE

Whenever your children, no matter what their age, do something that appears unusual, other knowing parents, grandparents and books on raising the 'perfect' child will all inform you that 'it's just a phase'.

Your parents remind you what a brat you were at that age — whichever age it is. Friends relay their experiences, the consensus being: 'There's nothing to be concerned about, it's just a phase.'

There are many phases, many different stages of development. Accompanying each developmental milestone are moments of great joy — the first word, the first step, the first school report card. But of course there are also times of distress, rage and panic — the first time the school calls to say your child has been suspended, the first time the police bring them home, the first time they scream, 'I hate you and I want to kill myself!', and the list goes on.

Adolescence, the phase of your child's life that no one can prepare you for — well, properly, that is —

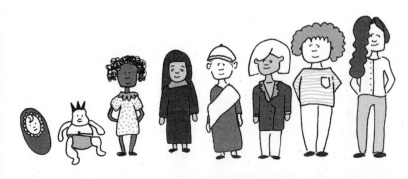

(some) STAGES OF DEVELOPMENT

is in fact a developmental stage that is considered to be a comparatively recent phenomenon. It is my observation that it is also primarily a first-world phenomenon.

HISTORICALLY . . .

In the Western first world, along with other Westernised developing nations, childhood and adulthood seem to have been pushed further apart. In the not-so-distant past, children were considered to have reached adulthood as soon as they were old enough to leave school and find work to support themselves.

Nowadays, the traditional roles and expectations for children and adults are less defined, and this can lead to confusion for both adolescents and their parents. Part of this is a result of social realities such as economic dependence — via student loans — and at times very limited employment opportunities.

Teens and young adults may be struggling with their gender identity and/or their sexuality. They are often experiencing exaggerated feelings of helplessness. Their frustrated attempts at achieving autonomy, self-determination and independence from the parental relationship can often lead to hopelessness and despair, emotions that provide a perfect host environment for depression and anxiety.

International research shows we are experiencing depression in epidemic proportions, and also alerts us to the trend towards more depression at a younger age — a trend verified by the increase in teenage suicide rates.

MY OPINION

I am certainly not about to argue with the stats on teenage suicides, nor am I arguing about the increasing rates of teenage depression. However, what I do present for consideration is that the true epidemic with our youth is *anxiety*.

I believe that young people get to the point where they can no longer deal with the constant battle with their internal critical dialogue (negative thoughts). These thoughts can often result in an overwhelming sense of physical and emotional discomfort.

As these thoughts continue to dominate, the internal world of thought becomes a battlefield of anxiety, self-doubt and a diminishing sense of worth. Finding themselves living in this distressing internal world, suicide appears to offer an escape.

The next section provides some background on my expertise in teenage mood disorders (and hence my unabashed delivery of my clinical opinion).

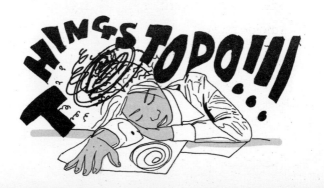

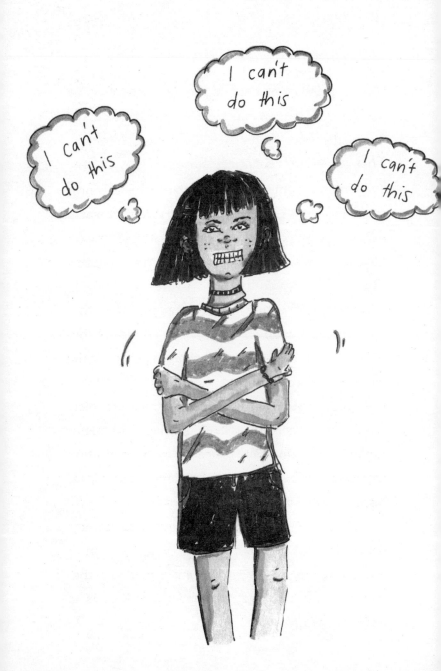

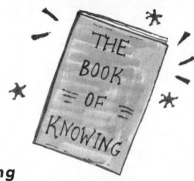

The Book of Knowing

This book was designed to explain to youth how to navigate their thoughts and emotions. It was a result of the demand I saw for a blog I was writing for distressed teenagers. I was subsequently swamped with teenagers in my clinical practice.

What became increasingly apparent was that they were not so much depressed as anxious. What research now tells us is that prolonged anxiety is the pathway to depression.

Rather than suicide being understood as solely a result of clinical depression, perhaps it is better explained as an intolerance of and frustration with ongoing anxiety, with at times a catastrophic response (suicide) to the discomfort.

Hence I believe that our approach to teenage depression needs to be initially an exploration of anxiety. Teenagers are no different to adults, in that their systems will also shut down in response to excessive strain.

WHY ARE YOUNG PEOPLE SO ANXIOUS THESE DAYS?

This is a question often asked by parents and by family members from the older generations!

There is no one reason, especially not within this new technological world. Young people live within an increasingly complex society, overflowing with prejudice, ignorance and intolerance.

Take bullying as an example. It is not that bullying is new — the playground has always been cruel — but now this cruelty can be spread with the touch of a button. Instantaneous viral humiliation. Now that's new!

Yes, there is social media, with its curated perfect lives and the subsequent feelings of inadequacy. But you cannot place the blame on one societal phenomenon. Because when you look closer, not every youth on social media experiences anxiety and/or depression. Hence, social media is not solely to blame.

'Is it nature or nurture?'

Neither, and both. There's no right and no wrong.

The scientific research that takes us a bit closer

to understanding ourselves, and our loved ones, is in the area of epigenetics. Epigenetics is the study of how your behaviours and environment can cause changes that affect the way your genes work.

So you can have a genetic predisposition to a particular condition. However, this is only considered a liability or a tendency. It doesn't necessarily mean you will develop it.

This leads us to the research findings that suggest anxiety has a genetic predisposition of 25-40 per cent — ridiculously high when you think about it, considering predisposition to cancer is estimated to be 5-10 per cent.

You may have given birth to a child with a hypersensitivity that is genetically predisposed. That means hypersensitivity to all things joyous and all things toxic.

This hypersensitivity usually accompanies them through their childhood and into their teens and young adulthood. We refer to this as 'temperament'. It is often evidenced by ongoing separation anxiety, shyness, worry and difficulty making friends.

Throw all this in a mix with a multitude of malignant environmental expectations and you

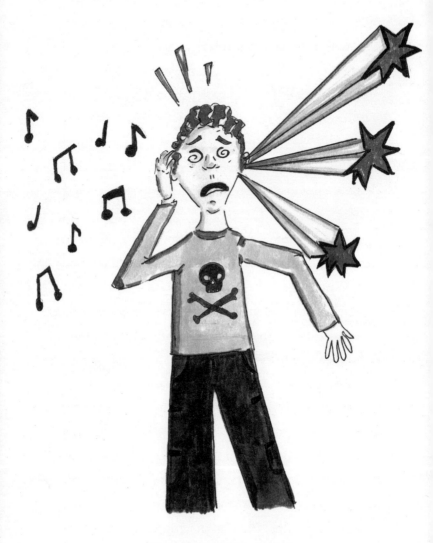

Hypersensitive children can feel
overstimulated by their environment.

begin to grasp the complexity of the bigger picture: a biological contribution, with social *and* psychological contributions.

Other factors

The onset of depression can often be linked to a close and significant bereavement in the family, particularly if there is a family history of depression. Other severe stressors include physical or sexual assaults.

Another theme that emerges in the teen and depression literature is the increased risk of suicidal behaviour in young people with poor self-esteem and aggressive or antisocial traits. Poor parent–child relationships, family dysfunction and family breakdowns are all identified as risk factors.

Puberty is an important developmental stage. Mother Nature pushes, via evolution, the primal need to be part of a group, find a mate and ultimately breed to maintain the survival of the species. However, in a binary-dominated world, this is not always as easy as it sounds.

Puberty is the stage for increased sexual awareness and issues to do with sexuality. Decisions are being explored with regard to sexual preference. Young people who are struggling with their sexuality can be very vulnerable to depression. They are at even more risk if they are in family or school environments where they could be fearful about the possible responses from their families and/or peers.

I will never forget this story from a gay man in his thirties, who after a cheeky glass of wine told me about his 'coming out' to his mother.

It took me a lot of courage, but I had decided that in order to be myself I needed to tell my parents that I was gay. My mother looked at me with revulsion in her eyes and said, 'I'd rather you had told me you have cancer.' She quickly exited and vomited, within hearing distance.

I don't think I have to detail the psychic damage this reaction had caused!

BACK TO THE 'JUST A PHASE' THEORY . . .

Something that often bewilders parents of teenagers is how to differentiate between this 'phase they are going through' and something more serious.

Their clothes are black, their music sounds black, and every time you won't let them use the car their mood turns black. So how is it possible to detect depression in your teenager, when so much of their behaviour looks to you like the ordinary teenage behaviour your friends and family describe? Are they sleeping a lot because they talk all night on the phone, or perhaps they are in the middle of another growth spurt? Or could it be the early onset of schizophrenia or depression?

Take a look at this symptom checklist, based on information from the World Health Organization. It could be helpful in clarifying your concerns.

Changes in weight or appetite

Adolescent eating patterns are difficult to assess, particularly with many teenage girls constantly dieting and the prevalence of eating disorders, increasingly in young males as well as young

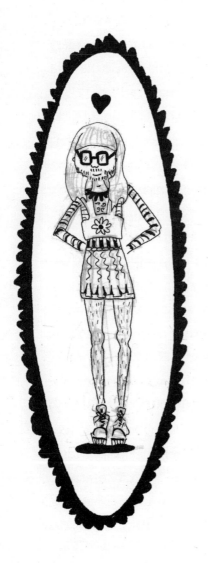

IT'S
NOT A
PHASE,
—————
IT'S
GROWTH.

females. Look out for stopping eating regular meals and changes in bodyweight of more than 5 per cent per month. (Note: If they have an eating disorder, they will try to hide their weight reduction.)

Constantly complaining of being bored, hating school

It is important to be aware of any marked changes in school performance — failing exams, refusing to go to school, etc. This could be happening as a result of bullying, but either way it needs to be talked about.

Feelings of sadness

Do these feelings last most of the day and are they present most days? Constant irritability and/or tearfulness can also be a sign.

Feeling guilty, hopeless or worthless

They may have a marked over-concern with the state of the world, especially given that this current generation are very aware of the environmental carnage taking place. They might be preoccupied with the world coming to an end, nuclear wars or climate change.

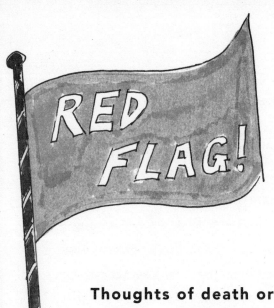

Thoughts of death or suicide

Constantly talking about death, only ever listening to depressing music, and idolising cult figures and celebrities who have taken their lives. There may be suicide attempts, and in particular a specific plan of how they would commit suicide. THIS IS THE BIGGEST RED FLAG.

Changes in sleep patterns

They might be watching screens all night because they can't sleep, or they might be in bed all day because they can't face the world.

Inability to concentrate, remember things or make decisions

Our conscious mind is a very limited piece of cognitive real estate. Hence, if the mind is full of worry and negative thoughts, executive functions such as memory and decision-making are quickly impaired. This can also manifest itself in changes in performance at school — as their concentration span decreases, so does their ability to achieve academically. (Note: Also consider the possibility of learning disabilities and/or attention deficit disorder being factors.)

Fatigue or marked loss of energy

Adolescence is a time of significant physical growth (which requires energy), so young people do tend to sleep a lot. The key indicator here would be a lack of energy to connect with peers or pursue favourite activities.

Loss of interest sexually

Your teenager may or may not be sexually active, but a complete loss of interest in the pursuit of romantic attachments is a sign to watch for.

Loss of interest or pleasure in activities they once enjoyed

This is especially important if you begin to observe them becoming socially more isolated. Adolescents can enjoy doing a lot of things that might seem annoying to you, so more often than not these activities will be saved for their friendship group. Hence, cutting off from their peer group is a very important indicator of depression.

And finally . . .

Substance abuse

Depression in teenagers is often accompanied by tobacco, alcohol and/or drug abuse, such substances of course being an immediate — although temporary — fix for anxiety. Most teenagers tend to experiment, but it is ongoing abuse that needs to be looked out for and subsequently addressed. It can also lead to promiscuous sexual behaviour, along with risk-taking behaviour such as driving while intoxicated.

Hopefully, the information in that checklist will help you to differentiate between 'teenage stuff' and possible depression. If you can tick off four or more of the described symptoms in your teen, I suggest you seek professional advice.

TYPES OF PROFESSIONAL INTERVENTIONS

Psychoeducation

This is a type of education focused on psychological issues, in this case depressive illness and treatment strategies. Wherever possible, this educational process needs to include the entire family, not just the person experiencing depression.

All family members are affected by living with a depressed individual, and discussions that promote understanding of the illness do serve to ease tension within the family environment.

Knowing more about symptoms and the early signs of recurrence of the illness will enable both the teenager and their family to seek the right treatment and help prevent relapse.

Pharmacotherapy (medication)

Young people are often very ambivalent about medication, but if the mood state is depression and not 'just a phase' medication plays an important part in treatment. When a medication is prescribed, ask for specific information on the choice of drug and any current research on its effects and benefits. If the family understands the purpose of the medication, they can help to make sure that it is being taken as prescribed.

It's essential to get siblings onside too, to prevent collusion with treatment resistance (not taking the medication). The siblings might be concerned about what is happening and not like the idea of their sibling being on 'drugs', so may encourage this non-compliance out of naivety.

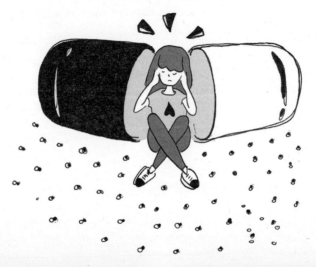

Hospitalisation

This is a very rare intervention, usually reserved for those who are psychotic or acutely suicidal, or who may have made repeated self-harm or suicide attempts. It is primarily for patients who cannot be managed at home.

Having your child hospitalised is a huge decision to make, so make sure you discuss it thoroughly with your mental health provider. Wherever possible young people need to be hospitalised in adolescent units, not with adults.

Psychotherapy

Both individual and family therapy play an important role. Individual talk therapy is essential in combination with medication. Family therapy sessions can provide an arena for the family to discuss and attempt to resolve the tensions and frustrations that result from the depression.

OTHER THINGS YOU
CAN DO TO HELP

Be there to listen

All human beings who feel sad need to have their feelings acknowledged by those close to them. If the 'snap out of it' approach or simply ignoring the problem worked, there wouldn't be a need to develop treatments for depression.

Encourage them to open up

You may have to invent creative ways of getting your loved one to open up, but it is important that you know how they are feeling. This is especially important if suicidal intent has been expressed. If you don't communicate openly, you will find yourself snooping through diaries and vetting phone calls. It is better to be able to talk directly, without judgement.

Help them to feel good

Try to remember something they used to enjoy and made them feel good. Maybe taking a long bath, going swimming, eating ice cream. Apart from

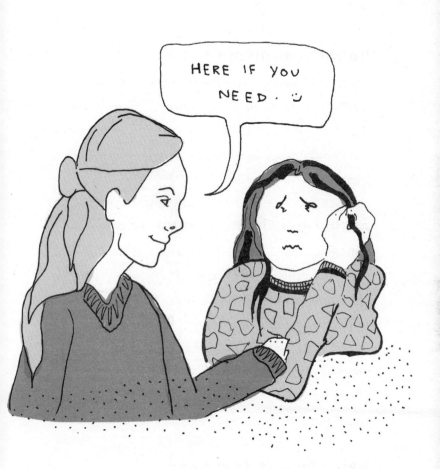

anything else, doing these activities will provide them with a distraction.

Encourage them to talk

Often teenagers will talk to anyone except their parents. Resist the temptation to interfere with this — in fact, encourage your teen to talk to others. However, a word of warning: if your teen is talking to your friends or other family members, insist that they let you know if there is any conversation about considering self-harm or suicide.

Ensure their safety

One of the most important things right now is that your child is safe. Clear medicine cupboards of pills or medications that could be used to overdose.

Lock away sharp objects such as knives and scissors, remove any firearms from the house, and in extreme cases lock away alcohol and cleaning products such as bleach and disinfectant. These final suggestions are extreme measures, but sometimes they need to be used.

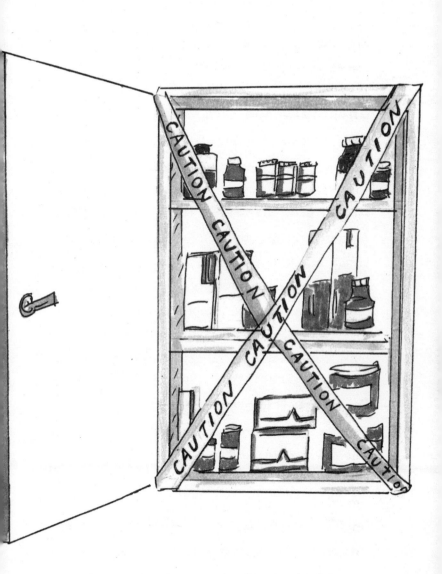

Try to help them with their decision-making

As a result of the depression and/or anxiety, they may be struggling with the simplest of decisions. Help them organise their daily activities. They may not be able to ask for help, so take the initiative.

Be a little intrusive if you have to

No teenager wants you to interfere with their friend group, but it is important that it is understood that things are not quite 'normal', and that even recreational drug use is not helpful at this time. Likewise, if you are observing them withdraw from friends, you may want to instigate contact.

Don't be frightened to ask

Talking and asking questions about your child's suicidal thoughts will be scary for you, but it is better that you know.

Don't forget other family members

Because your depressed child is your main focus at this point in time, your other children may be going through times of feeling left out and perhaps a little resentful. Their feelings need to be acknowledged, and they need to be kept informed about what is happening.

Get involved

Of course you want to respect your teenager's privacy, but you can request to be involved in appointments with mental health professionals. Insist upon both joint and individual sessions, and family therapy where necessary.

Don't forget yourself

Make sure you are taking time out for yourself. The role of caregiver is a stressful one.

Don't do the following

- blame yourself
- feel guilty
- go to sleep at night thinking 'Where did I go wrong?'

These things don't help!

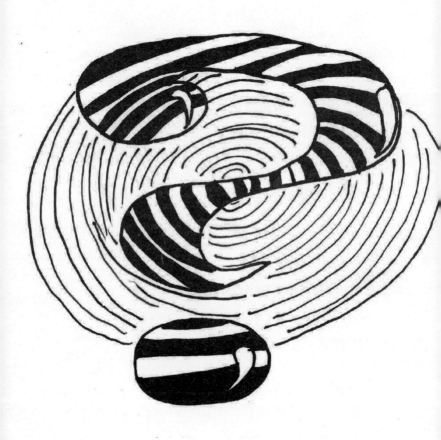

CHAPTER ELEVEN

GENDER, SEXUALITY AND DEPRESSION

If you have a family member or close friend from the rainbow community who you are concerned about because of their mood, this chapter is partly for you. And if you personally relate to the struggles in the pages to come, keep reading.

I was originally going to call this chapter 'Who would choose to be different?' This came from something I heard many years ago. During the AIDS epidemic of the 1980s, I was listening to a minister in San Francisco commenting on the refusal of the Catholic Church to administer the last rites to gay men dying of AIDS. His comment 'Who would choose to be different?' stuck with me. I thought to myself, 'Who would *choose* a life of discrimination, prejudice, injustice and contempt?' Hence, if there is no choice involved in sexual preference, then it must be biological, organic, genetic! I maintained that viewpoint for years, not realising that I had made a giant leap from nurture to nature.

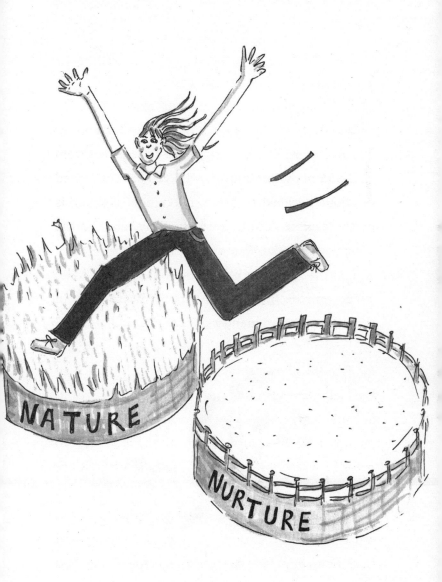

NATURE

NURTURE

In actuality, it is not an either/or situation. It is not absolutely about genetics, nor is it all about environment. It is about epigenetics, the interactions of both factors in unison. Hence the outcomes are like the colours of the rainbow, the diversity of a spectrum.

The relationship between biology and sexual orientation is a subject of much research. While scientists do not know what exactly determines sexual orientation, they theorise that it is caused by a complex interplay of genetic, hormonal and environmental influences.

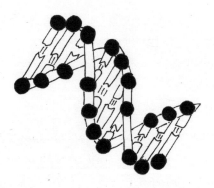

Finally, I got it! It is with this new understanding that I present you with my opinions on gender, sexuality and depression.

THE SEXUALITY SPECTRUM

The sexuality spectrum refers to the idea that our sexual identities and orientations are complex and resist easy classification, although they are often judged on the basis of their position between two extreme points. In the case of sexuality, for a long time it was considered a matter of right or wrong, good or evil, normal or abnormal — even as far as legal or illegal!

I really like the following synopsis from WebMD:

Instead of offering people a choice between either homosexual or heterosexual — or even a choice between homosexual, heterosexual, or bisexual — the spectrum provides a way of talking about sexuality in terms of many possibilities.

The sexuality spectrum also allows for greater fluidity of sexual identity and expression. Large-scale studies show that people often have sexual orientation ranges rather than fixed orientations.

For me, all of this research and debate merely emphasises the need for the acceptance of diversity — along with the realisation that we *all* coexist on a spectrum, for this is the essence of humanity.

Yet for the millions of our LGBTQI+ (lesbian gay bisexual transgender queer intersex) fellow humans, life is often not that easy. Why? Because as a species we have learned how to judge, to only feel comfortable when the world is seen in black and white — at either end of the spectrum.

Mother Nature doesn't operate within that paradigm. Probably her most well-known and admired spectrum — and my personal favourite — would have to be the beloved rainbow. It is no big revelation that a rainbow flag has become the emblem of the LGBTQI+ community and movement.

The original rainbow flag designed by artist Gilbert Baker featured eight horizontal stripes (see page 234), but the most common variant now has six. Many other pride flags have been developed to represent identities within the LGBTQI+ community — for example, the transgender flag and the progress pride flag, which appears in the background of the illustration on page 244.

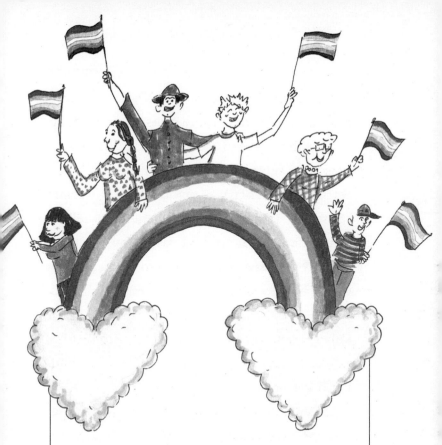

The story behind the rainbow

In 1978 the artist Gilbert Baker, an openly
gay man and a drag queen, designed the first
rainbow flag. Baker later revealed that he was
urged to do it by Harvey Milk, one of the first
openly gay elected officials in the US (a brave
man). He wanted to create a symbol of pride for
the gay community. Baker decided to make that
symbol a flag.

As he later said in an interview: 'Our job as gay people is to come out, to be visible, to live in the truth, as I say, to get out of the lie.' A flag really fitted his mission, because it was a way of proclaiming his visibility or saying, 'This is who I am!'

Baker saw the rainbow as a natural flag from the sky, but he adopted eight colours for the stripes, each colour with its own meaning:

- hot pink for sex
- red for life
- orange for healing
- yellow for sunlight
- green for nature
- turquoise for art
- indigo for harmony
- violet for spirit.

Now that palate of definitions is what I call an impressive, magnificent and wonderful representation of the multiple dimensions of life!

SOMEWHERE OVER
THE RAINBOW . . .

On the subject of symbols and emblems, let's look at another snapshot of this multidimensional community. The 1939 movie *The Wizard of Oz* became a haven and an escape, as well as a code in desperate times, for this alternative, non-conformist community. At that time, homosexual acts were illegal in the United States and in many other parts of the world. Stating that (or asking if) someone was a 'friend of Dorothy' was code for discussing sexual orientation without others (outside of the club) knowing its meaning.

Dorothy (played by Judy Garland) was the main character in *The Wizard of Oz*, wearing her ruby slippers and singing the inspirational song 'Somewhere Over the Rainbow'.

Judy Garland became an icon for the gay community. Not only did she star in this amazing technicolour vision of diversity, but also her own life paralleled the lives of many people struggling in the gay community. She died tragically in 1969 as the result of an accidental overdose of the barbiturates she had been prescribed for most of her life. Garland's story is sad, and so are the statistics on depression and suicide in the rainbow community. It is estimated that rainbow suicide rates are five times higher than the mainstream.

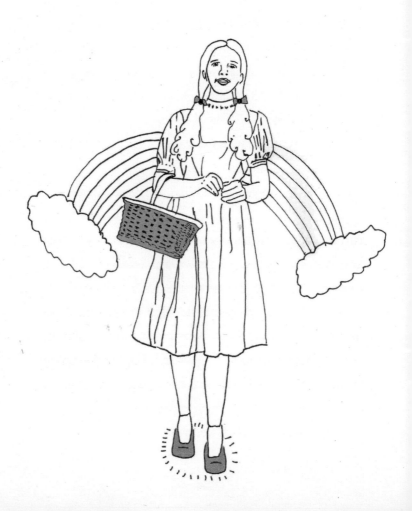

WHY ARE SUICIDE RATES SO HIGH IN THE RAINBOW COMMUNITY?

Well, here are a few clues:

- persecution for being different
- homophobia — within families, schools, communities and even doctors' and counsellors' offices
- rejection because you don't fit the 'norm'
- anger — your own or others' — at not being how you 'should be'
- fear of being attacked or murdered
- feelings of shame
- feelings of powerlessness and helplessness.

All of the above interweave and create a cold, dark and hostile climate in the mainstream world, far from the welcoming hue of the rainbow.

As a result of widespread homophobia, rainbow individuals of all ages describe feeling isolated, lonely and invisible. These of course are the types of feelings that can lead to depression, feelings of hopelessness and thoughts of suicide.

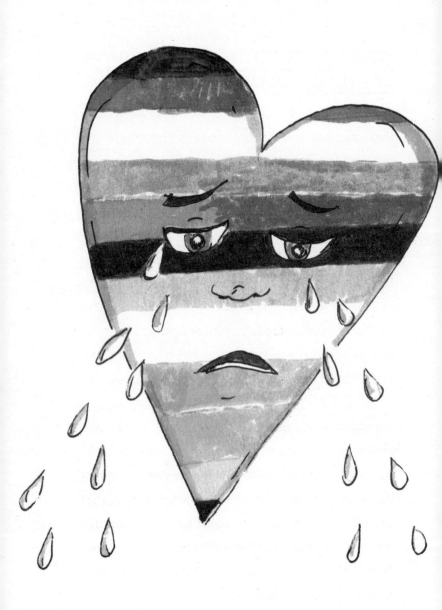

YOUTH SUICIDE IN THE
RAINBOW COMMUNITY

LGBTQI+ youth *do not commit suicide because they are gay*. Most consider suicide in response to bullying, discrimination, homophobia, depression, anxiety, substance abuse, violence, feelings of gender nonconformity, low self-esteem (often as a result of all of the above), and societal and family rejection, alongside conflict in relationships with regard to sexual identity.

The highest time of risk for suicide is when they first 'come out' to family and friends. The fear of a lack of support or of rejection by their loved ones and society drives this risk factor.

Pre-existing psychiatric conditions, as well as depression, anxiety and substance abuse, also create vulnerabilities.

For those who have been brought up to gain support and a sense of community from their church, religious doctrines can be very harmful if they condemn diversity of sexual orientation. These doctrines are also often damning of suicide itself, creating an impossible 'catch-22' situation.

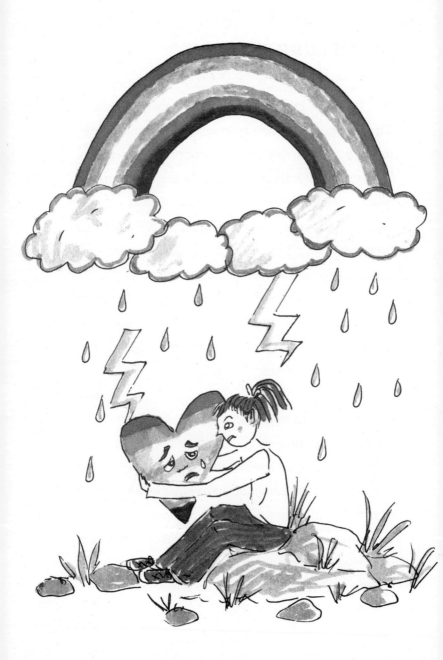

Be supportive

The number one thing is to support them by listening to and validating their experiences and feelings. Your response will set the stage for the outcome.

An embracing home environment has become especially important since the onset of Covid and home isolation, and since it has become more common for young people to remain living in the family home for longer. In fact, research shows that when LGBTQI+ youth have at least one accepting adult in their life, their risk of suicide decreases considerably.

It's important as a parent to understand that the future of LGBTQI+ youth can be just as brilliant and healthy as it can be for any youth, if you're being supportive and helping them be the person they can be.
— Myeshia Price (she/they), senior research scientist at The Trevor Project (www.thetrevorproject.org)

Emphasise that you love them unconditionally, and no less than their siblings.

Be flexible

Be supportive of wherever they're at, even if it changes over time. This is often a very fluid, transitional stage in their lives. Your support is more important than whatever the identity is.

Listen with empathy

Being supportive does not require mountains of knowledge, only a willingness to listen empathically.

Watch what you say, and how you say it

Pay attention to the language you use when talking about LGBTQI+ issues. This will improve with practice and guidance from your child. Avoid judgemental language; for example, 'You're too young to know what you are talking about,' 'You'll grow out of it,' 'You're just being rebellious and trying to hurt us!'

Being respectful of their wishes with regard to terminology, names and pronouns is also known to cut the risk of suicide. This is especially the case with transgender and nonbinary youth.

Let them be them

Give them space to be themselves; for instance, through their dress, mannerisms or choice of recreational activities and pastimes.

Take care of yourself

Acknowledge your own emotions. The focus when your child comes out is often on their feelings, but you will have feelings, too — some of which you may not feel totally comfortable with. You may find yourself experiencing a sense of loss for the future you imagined they would have, or disappointment about a potential lack of grandchildren. You may also fear for their wellbeing in the face of potential discrimination at school, in the workplace, wherever they may be in their lives.

Your friends and community may exhibit prejudices and ignorance, and so may also begin to isolate you as a family.

Find a way to express your feelings. You might want to try journalling or seek out support groups.

Important note: Try to process your feelings away from your child, so they don't end up feeling responsible for your distress and therefore think they must be doing something bad.

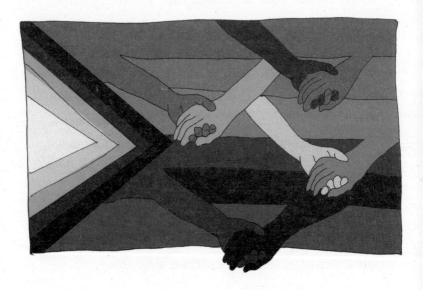

You're a family — keep being one.

IF YOU IDENTIFY AS LGBTQI+ . . .

Reaching out for help may feel somewhat overwhelming at first, but there is no shame in it, and nor is there shame in asking a friend or family member to make the initial call for you.

Be careful of where you go for an appointment. If you do not go to a therapist who is LGBTQI+ friendly, the therapy can risk being intrusive and ineffective.

When you first make contact, be upfront about wanting a therapist specifically skilled in working with the LGBTQI+ community. Don't be shy about enquiring as to their experience — any therapist worth working with will welcome the questions, knowing that for a therapeutic relationship to be effective the communication needs to be honest and forthright.

A way to ensure this connection is through the word-of-mouth recommendations of your peers. Support groups will also be able to recommend therapists. Such recommendations and resources are far more accessible now than ever before.

As with all therapy, when choosing who to work with and what type of therapy to engage with, consider the following:

- Be clear about your goals and what you want from a therapist. Are you looking for:
  * supportive counsel?
  * a diagnosis of a mental health condition, such as depression or anxiety, that may be a result of your struggle with your identity or sexual orientation?
  * professional guidance during your transition (if you are transgender)?
- You may be in a place where you are personally resolved with your sexual identity or orientation. However, the fear of rejection and/or rejection itself may still haunt you. A good therapist can help you navigate these difficult situations and assist in managing your anxiety.
- Make a commitment to yourself to work on building trust with your chosen therapist. Remember, it's not a game. It's not about being the smartest or the most complicated client ever and hence incredibly interesting!
- Don't forget you are in a high-risk group for depression, anxiety and suicide, so you need to take therapy seriously.

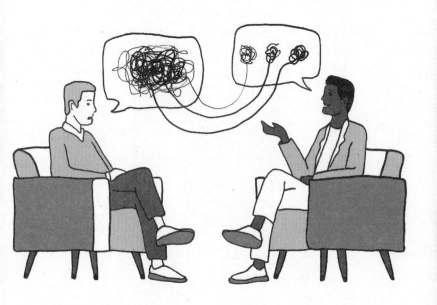

A good therapist can help you untangle the knot of issues you are dealing with. Make sure they understand what you want to get out of therapy.

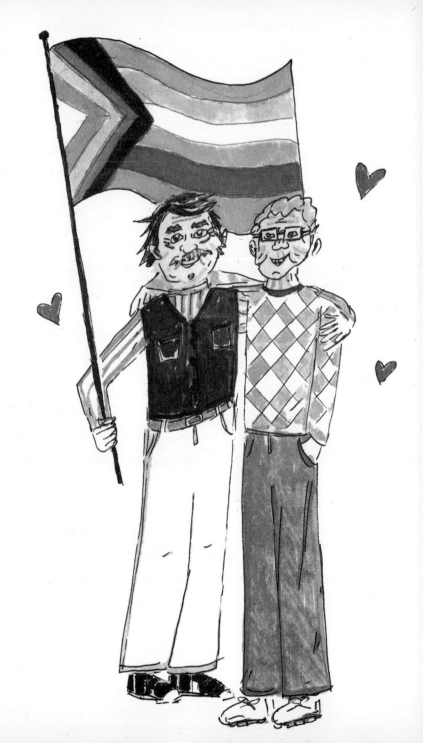

GROWING OLD UNDER THE RAINBOW

Chapter Thirteen (page 279) discusses depression in older people. However, in the LGBTQI+ community those in the older age group often experience unique fears and considerations. Among them are:

- Towards the end of life, when care is needed, will there be rest homes that are LGBTQI+ friendly?
- What other support might be available that is LGBTQI+ friendly?

This age cohort has usually had a very different experience of coming out than the younger people of today. They may have had a heterosexual marriage and raised a family before coming out, because that was the expected thing to do at the time.

I have worked with many women whose husbands announced their homosexuality much later on in life. The families usually end up divided and angry. The wives feel betrayed and bitter, and often make the following comment:

> 'If only he had had the guts to come out when I was in my forties or fifties — at least I would have had a chance to start a new life!'

However, way back then it was easier said than done. Those who choose not to come out often live a lifetime of regret and intimate solitude, well and truly caught between a rock and a hard place.

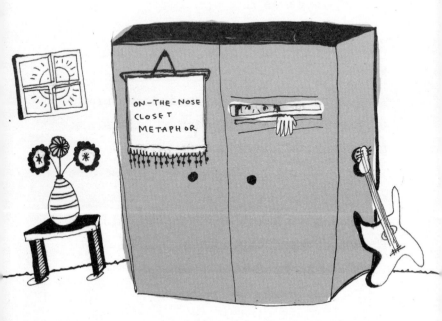

THE 'T' IN LGBTQI+

Transgender is another place on the spectrum that I thought I understood but didn't. Having primarily used the term 'transsexual', I had assumed that this was an issue of sexual orientation.

A dear trans friend of mine taught me that transgender has nothing to do with sexual orientation — it has to do with gender identity. Transgender is in fact a general term that describes people whose gender identity, or their internal sense of being male, female or something else, does not match the physical gender they were assigned at birth. It's a much more descriptive term than transsexual, as it makes it clear the issue is around gender identity, not sexuality.

I spent some time with my trans friend prior to compiling this chapter and learned the following from her personal experiences.

She recalled knowing she was different from the age of three — wanting to touch and play with fabrics, and not wanting to engage in the sporting activities enjoyed by her brothers.

Her mannerisms and body language tended to

be more 'effeminate'. Her childhood was plagued by constant bullying and harassment, to the point where she would walk to school rather than be subject to never-ending abuse from the others on the bus.

Not surprisingly, as a result of this discrimination, bullying and lack of acceptance, she grew up with anxiety and recurring depression. Shame was her constant companion.

A very determined human being, she fought to be the best that she could be at whatever vocation she chose to pursue. She looked for role models outside of the transgender stereotypes of the time — such as drag queens, substance abusers and sex workers — turning instead to successful people in other spheres.

When I asked her to summarise her experience of being transgender, she said quite simply:

'It was like my brain was in the wrong body.'

Over the years I have worked with the transgender community, I never cease to be amazed at how psychiatric conditions such as depression, anxiety and having suicidal thoughts can change almost immediately with the introduction of hormone therapy. It's almost like a miracle cure — a biochemical change that occurs.

That's all I have to say on the gender and sexuality spectrum — except to make the point that depression knows no boundaries. The depressive illness is oblivious to gender, race, age or sexual orientation.

If you are close to someone from the LGBTQI+ community, be kind, and make a point of opening yourself up to difference. Your experience of life will be richer, more colourful and a lot more fun.

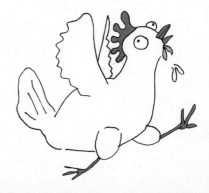

CHAPTER TWELVE

'WHY WOULDN'T I BE DEPRESSED?' — DEPRESSION IN CHILDREN

If your favourite grandmother had died,
if your best friend had moved away,
your sister had cancer & your dog had died.
You got bullied when you went to school . . .
how would you feel?
— A child

I think you and I both know how we would feel: very, very unhappy (to say the least). If we stayed that way for a period of time, there is a high probability that we would become depressed. Yet it doesn't seem to occur to us that children could suffer from depression, even though they are made from exactly the same raw materials as adults: mood receptors, a nervous system, stress hormones and so on.

In fact, it was considered so unlikely that there was not an official diagnosis for childhood depression until 1980, even though significant research had begun in the late 1950s.

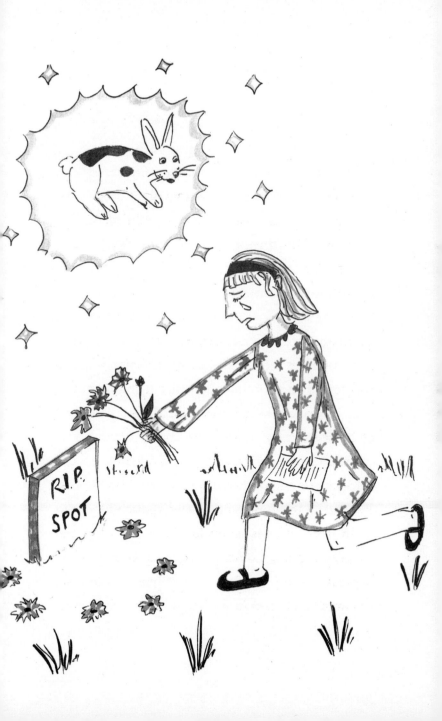

AN EYE OPENER OF A STORY . . .

In the 1950s, an American paediatrician — Leon Cytryn — was struck by the frequency of sadness and withdrawal that he saw in boys admitted to hospital for surgery on their undescended testicles. The prospect of this procedure is nothing to be happy about, I know, but the lowered mood was found to be not directly linked to the surgery itself.

Cytryn began to explore the emotional states of these boys, discovering that almost half of them had symptoms that would have been associated with adult depression: feelings of hopelessness, low mood, etc. He continued his research into the 1960s, and found many physically ill children to be markedly depressed. But Cytryn and his colleague Donald McKnew were aware that a diagnosis of childhood depression was not acceptable to the medical profession.

Medical teaching still insisted that children did not become depressed in a clinical sense. When McKnew tried to elicit help from other disciplines to study the biochemistry of these patients, no one was willing to co-operate. At that time the notion of childhood depression was deemed preposterous.

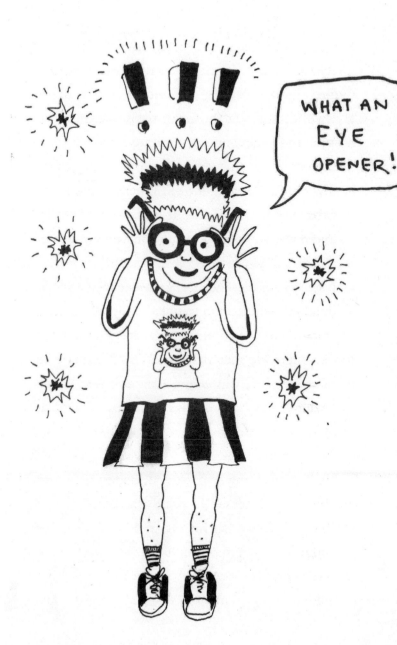

Fortunately attitudes have changed over time.

It is my clinical opinion that although society today is more accepting of adult depression, when it comes to children the belief set is still different. Some of the comments you hear are:

- The only people benefiting from all this talk about depression are the drug companies, and now they want to make money out of our children — it's outrageous!
- It's just a phase. They will grow out of it, and they will grow up stronger.

I'm not denying that there is a small element of truth in some of this scepticism, as there is still widespread academic debate about the diagnosis

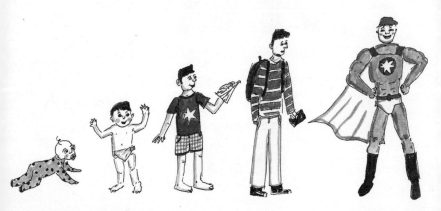

of childhood depression and about treating it with medication. However, what is no longer debated is the existence of depressive disorders in children.

Researchers are also now clear that depressed children are more likely to become depressed adults. I hear this in my clinical practice every working day:

When I really think about it, I don't ever remember being happy as a child.

HOW DO YOU KNOW IF YOUR CHILD IS DEPRESSED?

It certainly is not my intent to raise a false alarm and overdramatise a very natural response to sad and stressful events. However, the main point that I would make is that sadness is normal *in response to loss or grief.* There comes a time when it is no longer in context, and at that point your child is at risk of developing depression.

The following checklist, based on one shared by the World Health Organization, is a guide to knowing whether or not your child has crossed the line.

Is your child depressed? — a checklist

☐ irritability, low tolerance for frustration

☐ loss of pleasure in previously enjoyed activities

☐ frequent feelings of sadness

☐ overactivity or excessive restlessness

☐ frequent unexplained stomach aches, headaches and fatigue

☐ weight loss or failure to achieve expected weight gain (or, less frequently, excessive weight gain)

☐ consistent verbal expressions of sadness and hopelessness — 'I'll never feel happy again.'

☐ evidence of low self-esteem — 'The other kids at school are really bright; no one likes me.'

☐ frequent and excessive worrying, assuming that something bad is going to happen, that there will be a catastrophe, the family will get hurt

☐ changes in sleep patterns: difficulty falling asleep, waking in the middle of the night, or alternatively oversleeping and wanting to sleep during the day

☐ refusal or reluctance to go to school

☐ a marked drop in school performance, where previously they had been doing well

- ☐ little interest in playing with their friends
- ☐ decreased energy, often looking tired and moving slowly
- ☐ communication becomes difficult; speaking almost seems too much of an effort
- ☐ repeated thoughts about or attempts at running away from home
- ☐ unprovoked hostility or aggression, refusing to do things, getting into fights at school
- ☐ excessive tearfulness or frequently feeling like they want to cry
- ☐ morbid or suicidal thoughts, frequent fantasies about death and dying, repeated themes of death in drawings.

NB: No one symptom in this list equates to a diagnosis of depression or a clinically significant emotional problem. However, *any evidence of suicidal thoughts* must be taken seriously, regardless of frequency. If this happens, your child is in immediate need of professional help. It doesn't matter if it turns out that you have overreacted a bit — better safe than sorry.

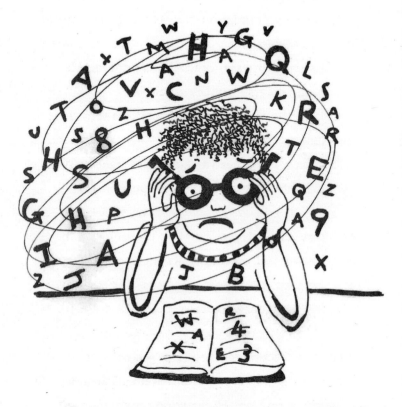

CHECK THIS BOX TO PROVE
YOU'RE NOT A ROBOT.

There are also other conditions that can mimic the symptoms of depression; for example, attention deficit disorder, post-traumatic stress disorder, learning disabilities and anxiety disorders. Hence an accurate diagnosis is essential.

Also worthy of note is that before these behaviours can be considered a symptom of depression, they need to be representative of *a change from how your child usually behaves*.

As I have said earlier in the book, the symptoms of lowered mood need to be present for more than two weeks, especially in the case of a grief response. However, depressed children will often not experience their symptoms consistently — they may come and go frequently and over a period of time. In their book *Help Me, I'm Sad*, David Fassler and Lynne Dumas recommend that parents need to concentrate on one key question when attempting to determine whether their child is truly depressed:

To what extent do your child's sad feelings and behaviour interfere with their everyday life and development?

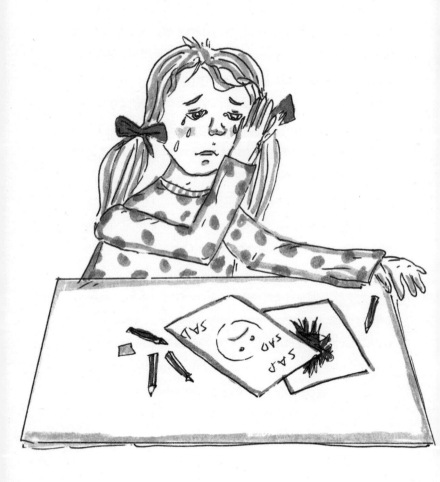

There are a number of measurement tools that can be useful in helping you to determine the answer to this question. The following inventory, which I like, can be used in either of two ways. You can answer the items yourself based on how you think your child would respond, or for slightly older children you could sit down with them and go through the questions, after suggesting it was something you were wondering about.

This inventory is a bit of a self-help test for you to use as an indicator, not as gospel — let the professionals establish the diagnosis.

The important thing here, as mentioned above, is to consider not only whether your child is experiencing these symptoms, but also how often and how much they are affecting your child's day-to-day life.

The Choate Depression Inventory for Children (CDIC)

[Answer **T**RUE or **F**ALSE]

		T	F
1.	I feel sad a lot of the time.	☐	☐
2.	I have trouble sleeping.	☐	☐
3.	I feel tired a lot of the time.	☐	☐
4	I don't have many friends.	☐	☐
5.	I cry a lot.	☐	☐
6.	I don't like playing with other kids.	☐	☐
7.	I don't feel as hungry as I used to.	☐	☐
8.	Other children don't like me.	☐	☐
9.	I feel lonely.	☐	☐
10.	I have lots of headaches and stomach aches.	☐	☐
11.	I don't like school.	☐	☐
12.	I have bad dreams.	☐	☐
13.	Sometimes I think about hurting myself.	☐	☐
14.	I worry a lot.	☐	☐
15.	I don't like myself.	☐	☐
16.	Other children have more fun than me.	☐	☐

17. I don't do as well at school as
    I used to. ☐ ☐
18. Sometimes I have a lot of trouble
    concentrating. ☐ ☐
19. I feel angry a lot of the time. ☐ ☐
20. I get into a lot of fights. ☐ ☐

NB: Answering 'true' for three or more items would warrant an evaluation by a professional. As mentioned earlier, a 'true' answer for item 13 — self-destructive, suicidal thoughts — always necessitates an evaluation.

TYPES OF HELP FOR CHILDREN

Children and adolescents with mild depression are usually treated with psychotherapy alone. If the depressive symptoms do not begin to improve within six to eight weeks, or if symptoms worsen, an antidepressant medication may be recommended. Before we go there, let's look at the therapy options.

Family therapy

The therapist works alongside the family, helping them identify relationship issues or communication difficulties that may contribute to the child's depressed mood. There may have been a lot of stress in the family or a significant death, and as each family member tries to cope with their own individual needs the communication links may have broken down.

A depressed child may actually be expressing some of the distress and symptoms of grief of the family as a whole. It is often more sensitive children who will manifest their unhappiness in this way. I call this being the carrier of the affect; in other words, the child manifests the often unsaid emotional climate of the family.

Family therapy is not designed to find blame, but is designed to develop more healthy ways of communicating, particularly when there are problems the family is dealing with.

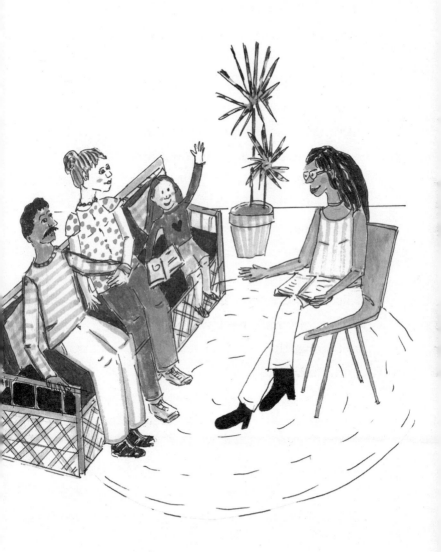

Individual therapy

Although family therapy can make a significant contribution, individual therapy for your child can also be essential. It is my clinical opinion that cognitive behavioural therapy (CBT) is very effective with children and offers a great deal.

The fundamental understanding of CBT is that depressed children, just like adults, can blame themselves when anything bad happens to them or their family (for example, the parents divorce). Children are even more prone to this because of the very nature of childhood — their state of being is very self-centred, meaning they feel the world revolves around them, so if something bad is happening, they experience it as being somehow connected to them.

CBT enables a process whereby the child's negative thinking can be identified. It also enables an identification of how the negative thinking patterns can contribute to changes in their behaviour. I love the way child cognitive psychologists will often use finger puppets to materialise the thinking patterns of the child, bringing to life the internal dialogue.

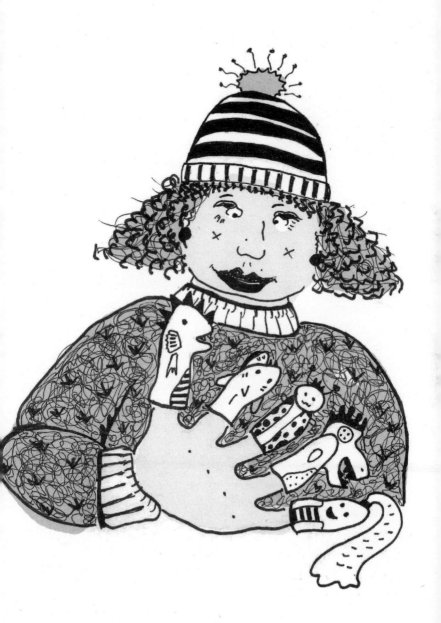

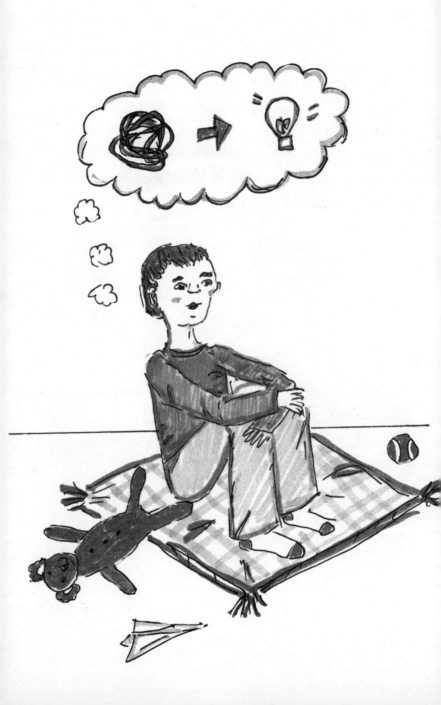

Once the themes of their thinking are identified, children are then equipped with skills to re-evaluate what is happening in a more positive (rational, non-emotive) light, and replace their self-defeating thoughts with more constructive and helpful ways of thinking, leading to more helpful ways of communicating and behaving.

Medication

There is still a lot of work to be done in the area of childhood depression, particularly in relation to the efficacy of medication. If your health professional recommends medication, ask lots of questions about its efficacy in children.

Although clinicians agree that medication should not be the first port of call, and nor should it be prescribed lightly or casually, medication can be extremely helpful and life-saving, particularly for children expressing suicidal thoughts. Medication is most helpful when the symptoms of depression you are observing are manifesting as a physical ailment, such as changes in appetite, low energy or trouble sleeping.

> Never allow your child to go on
> medication without a thorough
> medical check-up first. Be
> very aware of the similarity in
> symptoms between depression
> and other conditions, such
> as thyroid dysfunction.

Hospitalisation

In very, *very* extreme cases your child may need to be hospitalised. Care outside of the home is very rarely suggested. However, in cases where there is a risk of suicide, you may need to consider this as an option.

MY TOP TIPS FOR PARENTS

- You know your own child best.
- It will be *you* who observes any changes in behaviour and emotions.
- Check in with other people who know your child well, such as teachers, particularly given the role that bullying can play in childhood distress.

- Trust your instincts. If you have made sure there are no physical causes but you still feel something is wrong, consult a mental health professional — preferably someone with a specialist interest in children's mental health issues.

Ultimately, what you are doing is investing in your child's brain health, for both now and the future.

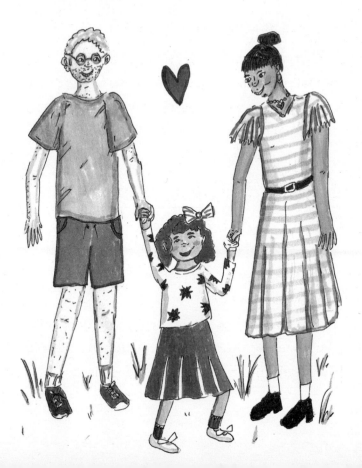

CHAPTER THIRTEEN

DEPRESSION AND OLDER PEOPLE

Old age ain't no place for sissies.
— Bette Davis, actress (1908-1989)

I find it fascinating how we perceive life as we pass through its various stages. I currently reside in the 'sunset' years of my life, as a late Baby Boomer (born 1955). I'm in that place in the theatre of life when there are no more dress rehearsals; when you've made your bed and now you have to lie in it; when you're reaping what you sow. However, old age isn't so bad when you consider the alternative. My favourite of the sayings that get bandied about is this one:

Inside every old person is a young person wondering what the f@#k happened.

Another fascinating realisation that occurred to me while I was writing this chapter is that I am in fact now statistically classified as 'elderly'. Clearly a

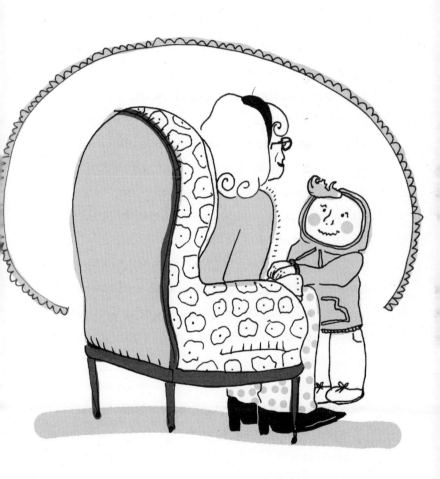

'GRANDMA, I'LL KEEP IT A SECRET
IF YOU SAY I'M YOUR FAVOURITE.'

perceptual oversight on my part!

Children don't really consider age that much until they are old enough to count the number of sleeps till their birthdays. Another wonderful thing about children is that they usually adore their grandparents, and their grandparents adore them. Being an actively involved grandparent can bring a lot of joy and purpose to life.

However, these happy stories do not apply to all grandparents. Young people learn that there are different groups of old people: there are those who give them a whole lot of stuff, cook wonderful food and want to kiss and cuddle them; and then there are the grumpy ones (perhaps from the other side of the family). They never seem pleased to see anyone and are never happy, just constantly complain about the noise.

Teenagers can be closer to their grandparents than their parents at certain stages. This is because clearly their parents have never been teenagers, and hence will never understand them, while their grandparents have always just been old!

As the unconditional nature of childhood passes, the vanity of young adulthood becomes the new

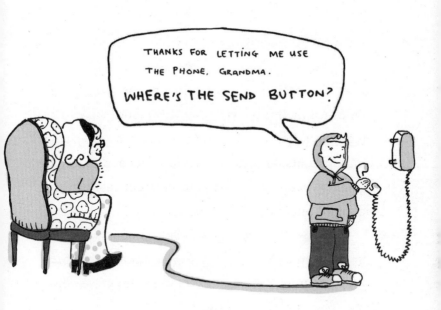

perceptual filter. They think that anyone who looks that old and has that many wrinkles would have to be miserable — particularly in the first world, where the pursuit of youth is a multi-billion-dollar industry, as the Baby Boomers race to defy 'looking old'.

It is not difficult to imagine that old age could be seen as an ongoing state of misery. Social outings tend to be catching up with friends and extended families at funerals, talking about the 'good old days', but never being quite sure whether they were good or not.

Even those of us with very full and active lives in the 'sunset years' will still have just below the surface a nagging fear of the reality of growing old alone. How will death arrive? Will it be kind and take you in your sleep, or will it be cruel and drawn out? Or will you lose your mind first? When you stop working, will you feel useless and redundant, anxious about your security?

It is such an uncertain and unknown territory. These very age-contextual fears are very often significant contributors to depression in the older age group.

MENTAL HEALTH AND AGEING

Societies that place no value on the contribution of their elders run the risk of worsened mental health outcomes for their older people. Older people do commit suicide, and the possibility should not be overlooked.

The following quote references undiagnosed depression in the older population.

Silent suicide is defined as the intention, often masked, to kill oneself by nonviolent means through self-starvation or noncompliance with essential medical treatment. Silent suicide frequently goes unrecognized because of undiagnosed depression and the interjection of the personal belief systems of health-care providers and family members.

Elderly individuals committing silent suicide are often thought to be making rational end of life decisions. However, the elderly committing silent suicide must be distinguished from terminally ill patients who refuse further treatment in order not to prolong the act of dying.
— Dr Simon Ri, *Journal of the American Academy of Psychiatry & the Law*, 1989

Of course both physical and mental health are dramatically affected by the very natural process of ageing. For example, older people might experience some of the following:

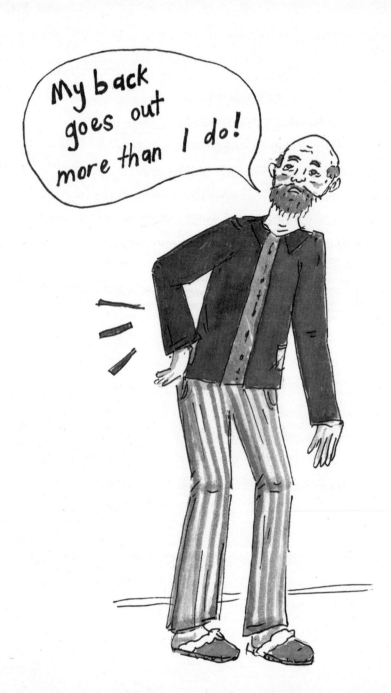

- hearing loss
- arthritis, back and neck pain
- cataracts and vision loss
- dementia and depression
- profound hormonal changes.

The other thing is that as we age, we are more likely to experience several conditions at one time — which may make it almost impossible for family members to be clear about what exactly is happening with an elderly relative.

Certainly old age is a time of great loss, both biologically and emotionally. However, the view that depression is a normal part of ageing, as well as being rampant in old age, is a myth.

In short, as an older person, if you are feeling down and lacking enjoyment in life most of the time, don't hesitate to go to your doctor. There is nothing that says you have to feel this way just because you are getting older.

INFORMATION FOR CAREGIVERS

For family members reading this chapter, the same applies. There is nothing to say that because your parents are ageing they will 'of course' be miserable.

As a loved one, often an adult child, you are most likely to be left with the responsibility of making all sorts of difficult decisions about your parents' health, and being constantly vigilant for unexpected physical and cognitive changes. Be aware that the family doctor may focus solely on the physical complaints and not explore the possibility of depression. This is not uncommon, particularly given the sometimes multiple physical ailments present. Of course, these conversations can also be easier to address than depression.

However, given that most older people with depression are Baby Boomers, at least awareness of mental health issues is higher than it was in the generation before them.

Navigating the complexity
of symptoms

Even if your parent(s) complain of terrible stomach discomfort or aches and pains, the symptoms of depression can still be identified by an expert. Certain GPs specialise in working with the elderly, but if this is not the case in your circumstance, seek out a geriatrician or a psycho-geriatrician who works with specific psychiatric and psychoneuro-logical (brain) disorders.

Specialist guidance is important, as it is very difficult to tell the difference between the symptoms of physical conditions and depression, especially when dementia is also involved. Depression and dementia can look very similar at the time of onset: in both cases the person slows down and there is a loss of enjoyment of life, as well as concentration and memory difficulties.

Depression can also be common in the early stages of such disorders as Parkinson's, or after a stroke, so thorough assessments are vital. But even if the depression is secondary to another condition, it is still important that it is treated.

Some signs to look out for

- losing interest in activities and interests
- preferring to stay at home rather than go out and do new things
- appearing to be constantly worried/anxious that something bad might happen to them
- not seeming happy, and lacking in energy, even for their favourites — the grandchildren
- pessimism about the future
- complaining of being bored (or having nothing to look forward to)
- a sad or depressed mood, expressing wishes to be dead
- not eating or drinking
- dramatic changes in sleep patterns.

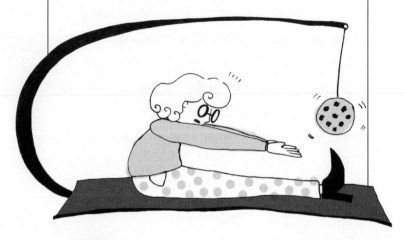

Clearly, you cannot know the extent of these issues without saying something out loud, so here are some questions to ask them, taken from clinical tools for the diagnosis of geriatric depression:

1. Are you still OK and satisfied with your life?
2. Do you often feel helpless, or that your life is empty?
3. Are you bothered by thoughts that you can't get out of your head?
4. Would you say you were in a good mood most of the time?
5. Do you feel you have a lot more problems with your memory than usual?
6. Do you feel worthless and that your situation is hopeless?
7. Do you think most people your age are better off than you are?
8. Do you get upset over little things and feel like crying more than you used to?
9. Do you have trouble concentrating and remembering, and feel like crying because of this?
10. Is motivation difficult, and you find yourself preferring to avoid social situations?

From experience I know these are difficult questions to ask and hear the answers to, even if asked by a professional. It is not easy to face the possibility that your parent or elderly loved one is depressed or wants to end their life, but it is better that you know and can begin the process of getting specialist help.

As I mentioned earlier, the elderly are often reluctant to have anything to do with 'mental health' issues. You may have to express your concerns to a doctor first, then take advice on how to encourage the person to attend an appointment.

If medication is recommended

The choice of medications, such as antidepressants or anti-anxiety agents, is dictated by the presence of other possible medical or surgical conditions, but these decisions are not medically difficult. The first choice for older adults is probably one of the SSRIs (selective serotonin reuptake inhibitors), which are heart friendly, don't alter blood pressure a great deal, don't compromise cognition (thinking processes), and compromise reaction time a lot less. They are not a risk for overdose attempts, but do keep an eye out for side effects such as agitation.

Other approaches

- Education about depression is important, for both the person suffering and their family.
- Cognitive therapy can be useful for non biologically-based negative thoughts.
- In the 65–80 age group it is not uncommon for the patient to prefer psychological and natural therapies to orthodox medication. If this is the case, discuss with their medical practitioner.
- Offer reassurance. Be kind — say you love them and you are there to help. Emphasise that you do not see them as a 'burden', which more often than not they will be thinking and feeling.
- Keep them occupied, and hence distracted from their psychic distress.

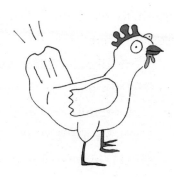

THE BURDEN OF CARING

As I mentioned earlier, often older people will feel like a burden to the family. This is a topic that is often not discussed — it is as though the burden of care is a well-kept secret.

In my opinion, it is often not spoken about because the family think they *should not* be feeling burdened or resentful about caring for their elders, who are loved and adored. Well, that may be the case in the *ideal* world, but in the real world taking care of a loved one — particularly if there are concurrent conditions such as dementia and physical poor health — is an emotionally painful, exhausting and at times unbearably frustrating time.

You are confronted with the vulnerability of someone you may have looked up to for the whole of your life, which can also raise your own sense of mortality and human fragility. So remember:

- Don't try to do everything on your own — network into as many support systems and professional resources as you can.
- There are many agencies that can offer respite care when needed.

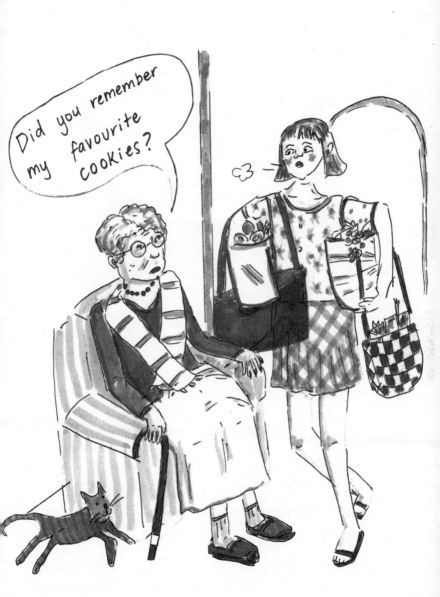

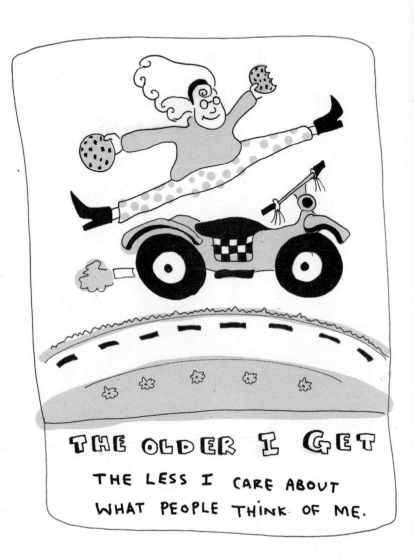

THE OLDER I GET

THE LESS I CARE ABOUT
WHAT PEOPLE THINK OF ME.

- You are allowed to feel frustrated at times — it doesn't mean you have stopped loving them.
- People do get tired of living at times, and that's life. But old age is not about being preoccupied with death — that's depression.

In the sunset of my life, I'm OK with my smiling lines AKA wrinkles. I'm happy with my wisdom, and I'm especially keen on not giving a f@#k about what other people think.

CHAPTER FOURTEEN

DEPRESSION —
A FAMILY AFFAIR

Depression is without doubt a 'family affair' in more ways than one. Let me explain . . .

Firstly, let's revisit the genetic predisposition for depression within families. Research puts the genetic contribution at between 15 and 20 per cent. For major depressive illness, in some studies the figures climb to as much as 50 per cent. Hence, when speaking with mental health clinicians about your own depression or that of a loved one, it is important to mention the family tree.

This enables your practitioner to determine whether or not the depression is in fact genetically predisposed. In my years of working with psychiatrists, I have not observed that this factor makes a great deal of difference with regard to the choice of medication — it is of interest to your practitioner, but it won't change what is prescribed. There is no drug which is specifically recommended for the treatment of depression that runs in families!

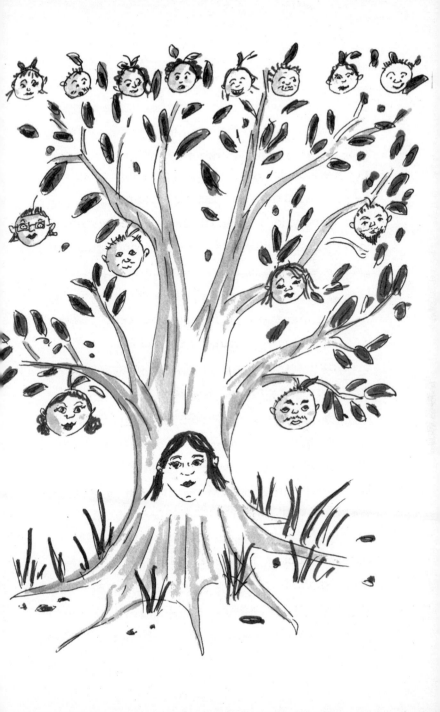

NON-GENETIC FACTORS

Refer back to what I said earlier about the study of epigenetics (page 207) to remind you about how your behaviours and environment can cause changes that affect the way your genes work.

Dysfunctional family systems are recognised to play a major part in depression both in childhood and adulthood. Severe childhood physical or sexual abuse, emotional and physical neglect, loss of a parent early in life, bullying, etc., can all be significant factors. Adults in the family can suffer from postnatal depression as well as depression as a result of all sorts of environmental strain: work, finances, divorce. I would also like to reiterate my observation that anxiety often has a very profound relationship with the onset of depressive illness. Hence, everyone in the family can be susceptible to experiencing depression — and some more than others — for all of the reasons we have explored throughout this book.

Not only is the existence of depression a family affair, but it is best managed that way, too. You may feel that your situation is unique and that you are to blame for being depressed, but you're not.

Because of the stigma surrounding depression, those who suffer from it and their closest supporters will often not want to discuss it beyond — or even within — the family. This means they can be reluctant to reach out for help and support, worried about what other people might think.

If that resonates with you, as either a depressed person or one of their supporters, remind yourself of the following.

- You don't know what other people are thinking.
- It is only your assumption that they are thinking judgementally.
- If it is a fact that they are thinking judgementally, f@#k them! You don't need that.

Talking, explaining, sharing emotionally and providing understanding — for *all* members of the family, no matter how young or old — is essential. This is how everyone will heal.

Depression isn't new —
talking openly about it is.

DON'T
FORGET
THE
LITTLE
ONES

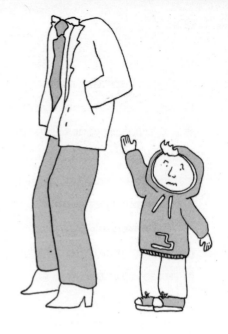

It's the easiest thing in the world to not include the children in all of this talking, depression often being considered a topic only for the young adults and grown-ups. You know how sensitive your children are — well, this sensitivity also applies when one of the family members is unwell. Hence, not explaining things to them can be frightening — far more frightening than an explanation.

They will know that something is wrong, but they won't know what it is. And the longer the silence is maintained, the more confused they will become. Eventually they may also start to feel that they are somehow responsible.

If you're wondering how to explain depression to a child, in her book *How Do We Tell the Kids?* author Pinky McKay offers this suggestion, which I think is lovely:

> *Depressed people are very, very sad. They may want to sleep a lot. Sometimes their illness saps all their energy so they can't play with you or talk to you. This doesn't mean they aren't interested in you anymore, or that they don't love you. The doctors will give them treatment to help them get their energy back and they'll be able to be happy again and join in with family activities.*

You will be able to put this into your own words, but the basic sentiment and content is there for you.

McKay also emphasises the importance of support and honesty to help children cope with a family member's illness. It is also worth considering that children can be quite cruel to each other, and even at a young age they can carry prejudices surrounding mental illness.

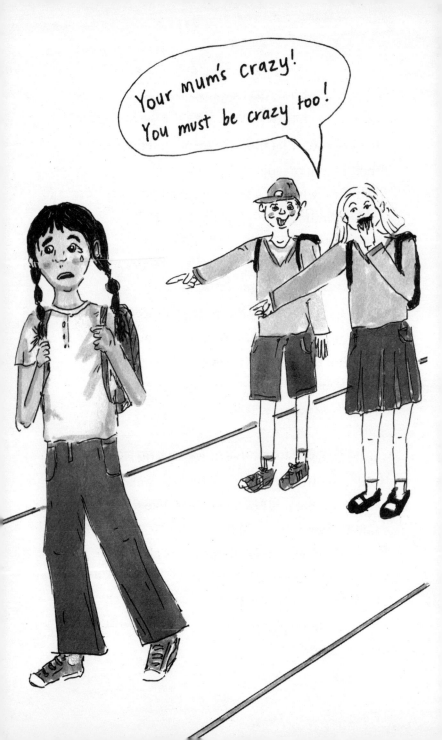

Children need to be equipped with the right information to help them navigate such situations. Let them know that they don't have to tell other kids if their parent or elder sibling is unwell.

The following are a few more great pointers from McKay's findings:

- Depression can be described as 'emotional pain'. Emphasise that it is an illness, it's just that you can't see it. It is not about not caring.
- Children need to know they didn't cause it, and nor can they make it go away.
- Avoid making false promises about exactly when the illness will be gone.
- Explain to them what sort of doctors psychiatrists are, and perhaps how they are different from the family doctor.
- Explain that it is not contagious, like mumps or measles.
- As always, encourage them to talk about their feelings, fears and concerns.

Little people's feelings matter too — remember it's a family affair.

CHAPTER FIFTEEN

YOU'VE GOT A FRIEND

Whenever I think of this phrase I remember in my mind's ear the music and lyrics of Carole King's wonderful masterpiece of the same name. King's song talks about being there for someone anytime, no matter what.

Hey you — yes you, the friend. Give yourself a great big hug. It takes a lot of tolerance, love and understanding to support a depressed friend. You need to have a very strong commitment to the friendship for it to survive, often for many months, while the person is unwell.

There will be times when you feel that nothing you are doing offers the slightest bit of help; that nothing you say seems to make a difference. You are doing your best, and yet at times you feel as if you are not getting through.

Are you 'doing the right thing' when you listen to them talk about how they are feeling? Or perhaps you 'should' just tell them to get over it? Should you be doing more, doing less? Or maybe just doing something completely different? What a powerless position to be in! Hence the reason why friends and loved ones can often experience the vicarious and potentially contagious nature of depression.

When people are depressed — and I speak from experience — one of their biggest fears is that they will lose friends because they are dull and boring and morbid, and seemingly endlessly non-appreciative. However, talking from the inside of a depressive illness — as I can do — I know that they need friendship more than ever. I used to appreciate every moment I spent with a close and dear friend. From one who knows, the best thing you can do for your depressed friend is just be there — whip up the odd pasta or cheese on toast if you can, or order in. Just be yourself.

HOW MY FRIENDS COPED

The following are excerpts from conversations I had with a few of my dear friends, who found their own ways of helping me through what was to be a long and cold journey back to health. I feel confident that you will find something among these words of wisdom and kindness that will help comfort your very dear friend. For they *are* suffering, and they *do* need you, even if sometimes they try to tell you they don't.

Raine

I always felt that it was important to be supportive and reassuring. Depression seems to take away people's ability to cope — they are no longer able to cope with life's everyday setbacks without being totally flattened.

I tried to offer the reassurance that getting well takes time, that you have to face one day at a time and put one foot in front of the other.

Most of all, I think it's making yourself available, just being there to talk through things, with no expectations. The other thing is that as a friend you are able to be there and give the family a break.

Just like when you eat an elephant, you can only do it one mouthful at a time.

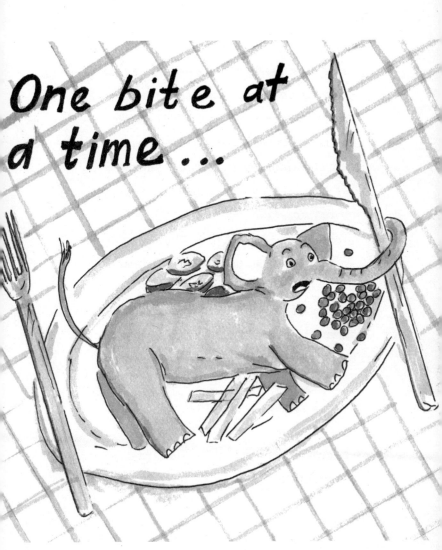

Donna

I used to think that being depressed was just being a bit low, feeling weepy and unable to control your emotions, and that the mood passes and you just snap out of it. I wasn't sure what to do at first. The worst part for me, as a friend, was not knowing what was going on and what to do.

I felt that it was important to try to bring things back to normality in some way — in a subtle way, like having close friends at home, rather than socialising amongst strangers, and to try to encourage a process of slowly re-emerging.

I couldn't agree more: human contact is fabulous, but not in large amounts — it's too overwhelming.

Kathryn

I don't know enough about depression or psychiatric illness to jump to the conclusion that my friend is unwell. It's almost as though, if it's a friend, you don't want it to be a mental illness. I would have to say that it was an acute learning curve for me. I've been able to see more things in hindsight.

I remember Kathryn seeming somewhat distant, because she was unsure of what to do and primarily wanted professional help to take over.

On reflection, I totally understand her position. Because someone you care for is depressed, you don't have to immediately rush in and be there at the front line — you can be there in the same way you have always been. Perhaps a little more, but only if it feels right. Don't offer help because you feel obliged — it won't work for either of you. Sending flowers and saying you care may be just what the doctor ordered.

Just remember: Being there is the most important thing of all.

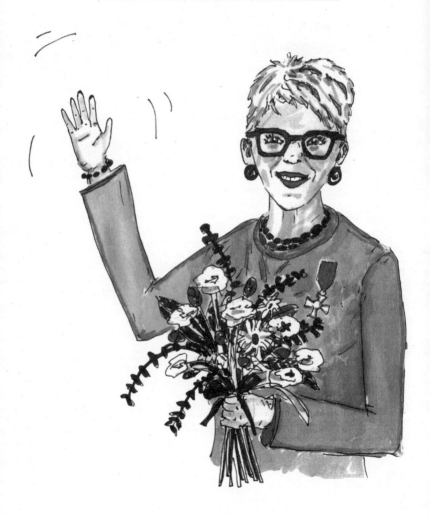